NO GALLBLADDER
DIET COOKBOOK AND FOOD LIST
FOR SENIORS

*Easy and Delicious Recipes and Foods to Eat for a
Healthy Gallbladder for the Elderly*

MARTHA J. KELVIN

Disclaimer:
The information provided in this book, is intended for educational purposes only. It is not a substitute for professional medical advice, diagnosis, or treatment. Always seek the advice of your physician or other qualified healthcare provider with any questions you may have regarding a medical condition.
The author and publisher of this book have made every effort to ensure that the information provided is accurate and up-to-date at the time of publication. However, medical knowledge and research are constantly evolving, and information may become outdated or subject to change. Therefore, the author and publisher do not warrant or guarantee the accuracy, completeness, or timeliness of the information presented in this book.
The author and publisher shall not be liable for any direct or indirect damages or injuries arising out of the use, interpretation, or application of any information provided in this book. Readers are encouraged to consult with their healthcare providers for individualized advice and recommendations based on their specific medical conditions and needs.

By reading this book, you acknowledge and agree to the terms of this disclaimer.
Printed in the United States of America.

First Edition: February 2024

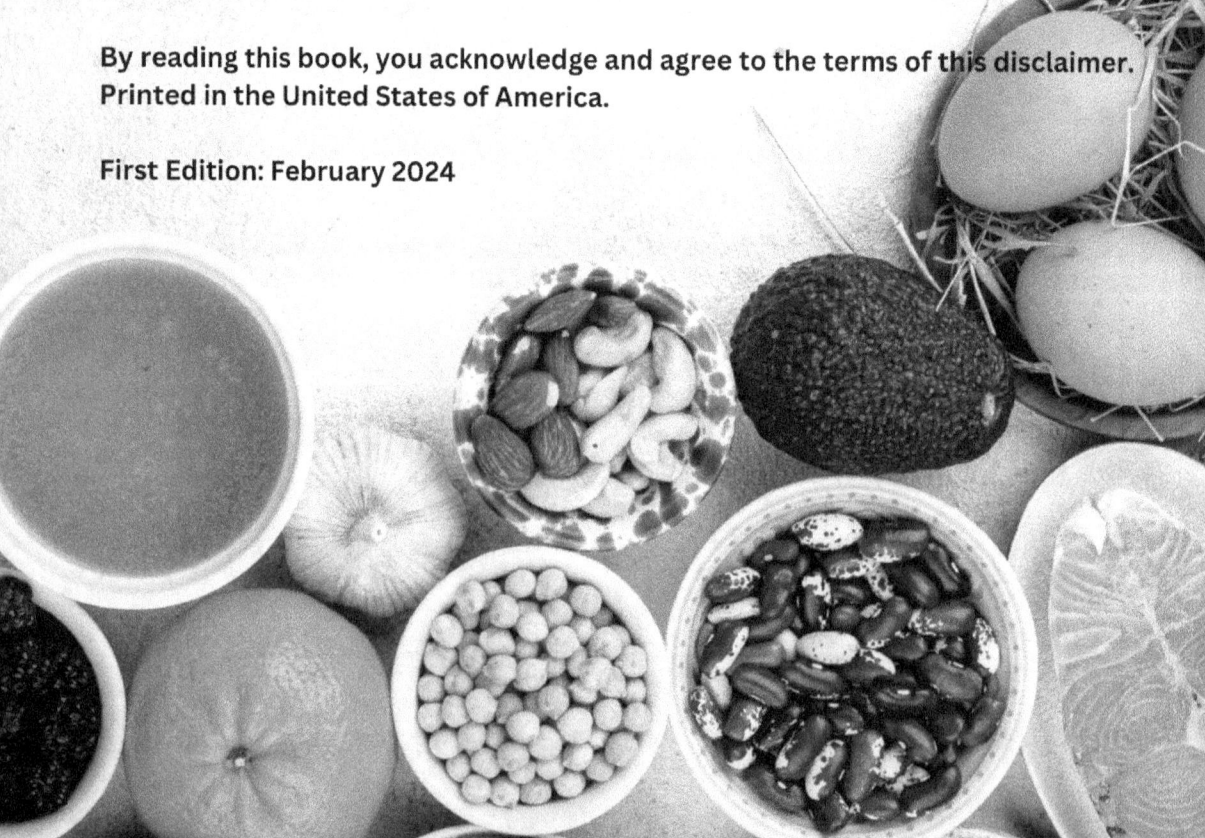

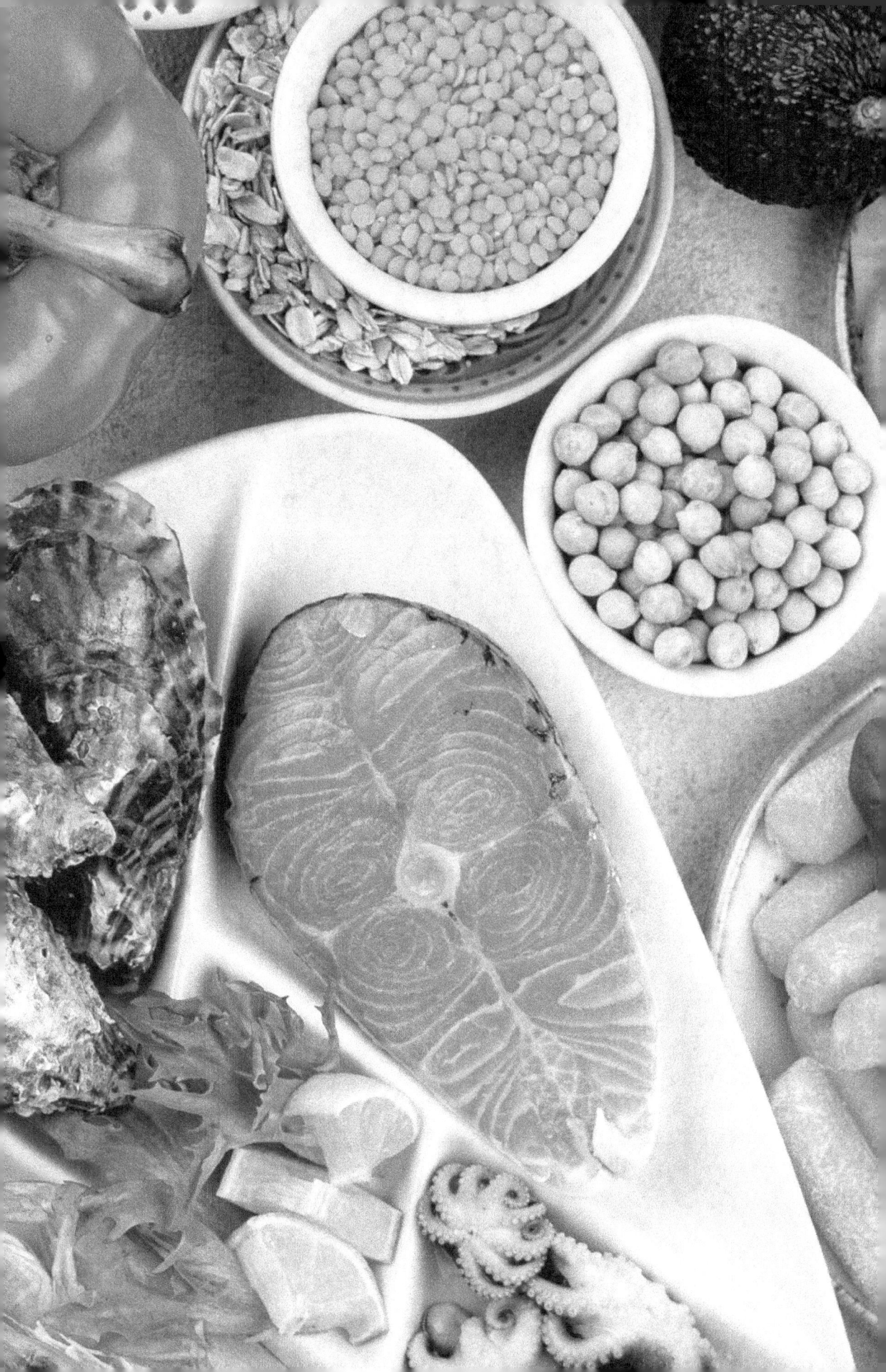

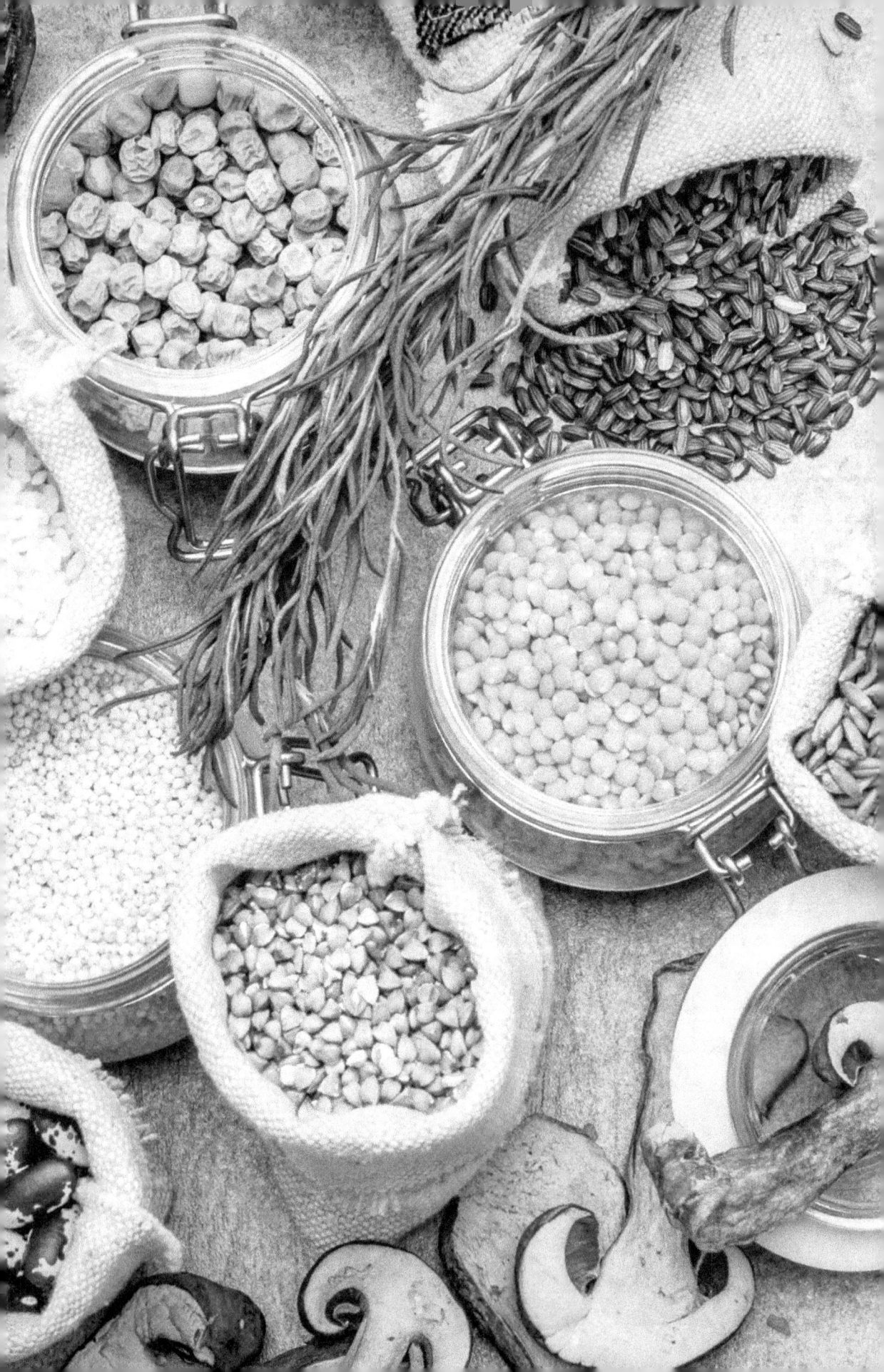

CONTENTS

INTRODUCTION

Cecilia's mornings began with the soft, golden light of Los Angeles seeping through her bedroom window, promising a new day, yet her body didn't share the same enthusiasm. At 67, she found herself grappling with a gallbladder that seemed to have its own, rather inconvenient agenda. This wasn't the retirement she had envisioned, one where her biggest concern should have been whether to attend a yoga class or meet friends for coffee, not navigating a diet that felt more like a minefield.

Her daughter, Jane lived just a few blocks away. Jane's visits were the highlights of Cecilia's week, bringing with them the chaos of work stories, dating mishaps, and the latest city gossip. Yet, recently, their conversations had shifted from light-hearted banter to discussions about fiber intake, the merits of turmeric, and the latest findings on gallbladder-friendly diets.

One particular Thursday, as Los Angeles basked in an unusually crisp morning, Cecilia found herself sitting across from Jane at their favorite breakfast spot, a cozy diner that had seen better days but held an irreplaceable spot in their hearts. The menu, once a source of comfort, now served as a reminder of Cecilia's dietary restrictions. She sighed, tracing her finger along the options, mentally crossing out items she could no longer enjoy.

Jane, ever the problem-solver, had come prepared with a list of gallbladder-friendly foods she had researched the night before. "Mom, did you know that beets are good for your gallbladder? And we can still have your beloved avocado, just in smaller amounts," she said, her voice a mix of enthusiasm and care.

Cecilia smiled, touched by her daughter's efforts. "I suppose this means we're becoming those people who discuss bowel movements over breakfast," she joked, trying to lighten the mood.

Their laughter filled the diner, a sound so familiar yet so precious. It was moments like these that reminded Cecilia of the strength of their bond, a bond that not even the most stubborn gallbladder could weaken.

As they navigated this new reality, their roles subtly shifted. Jane found herself worrying about Cecilia, her mother's health becoming a constant backdrop to her own bustling life. Meanwhile, Cecilia, who had spent a lifetime caring for others, had to learn to accept care, to lean on Jane not just for emotional support but for practical help in managing her condition.

Their journey was not without its challenges. There were days when Cecilia felt overwhelmed by the limitations of her body, and nights when Jane lay awake, fearing what the future might hold. Yet, through it all, they discovered a new depth to their relationship. Cooking together became their new therapy, experimenting with gallbladder-friendly recipes that didn't sacrifice flavor for health. They laughed at their culinary misadventures and celebrated their successes, finding joy in the simplicity of shared meals.

As Cecilia and Jane's culinary adventures unfolded, they stumbled upon a treasure trove of knowledge and flavors that transformed their understanding of food and health. Their journey, initially fraught with restrictions and uncertainties, gradually became a celebration of creativity and well-being. It was during one of their Sunday meal-prep sessions, surrounded by an array of colorful vegetables and the aroma of simmering spices, that Jane proposed an idea.

"Why don't we call Martha and compile our recipes and learnings into a book? Think about it, Mom. 'No Gallbladder Diet Cookbook and Food List for Seniors.' It could help so many people who are in the same boat as you," Jane suggested, her eyes alight with excitement.

Cecilia, initially taken aback by the idea, warmed up to it as she considered the potential impact. They had, after all, navigated through a maze of dietary advice, experimenting and learning what worked best for a gallbladder-less life. The thought of sharing this knowledge, of turning their personal struggle into a beacon of hope for others, was both humbling and exhilarating.

Together, they embarked on the task of compiling their recipes, each dish a testament to the love and resilience that had seen them through Cecilia's health challenges. They included personal anecdotes, tips for managing a gallbladder-friendly diet, and insights into the nutritional needs of seniors. The book was more than just a collection of recipes; it was a narrative of their journey, a guide infused with warmth, humor, and the wisdom gleaned from their experiences.

"No Gallbladder Diet Cookbook and Food List for Seniors" became more than just a culinary guide; it was a source of comfort and inspiration for those navigating the complexities of life without a gallbladder. For readers, it offered not just recipes, but a new perspective on health and well-being, emphasizing the importance of a supportive community and the strength found in shared experiences.

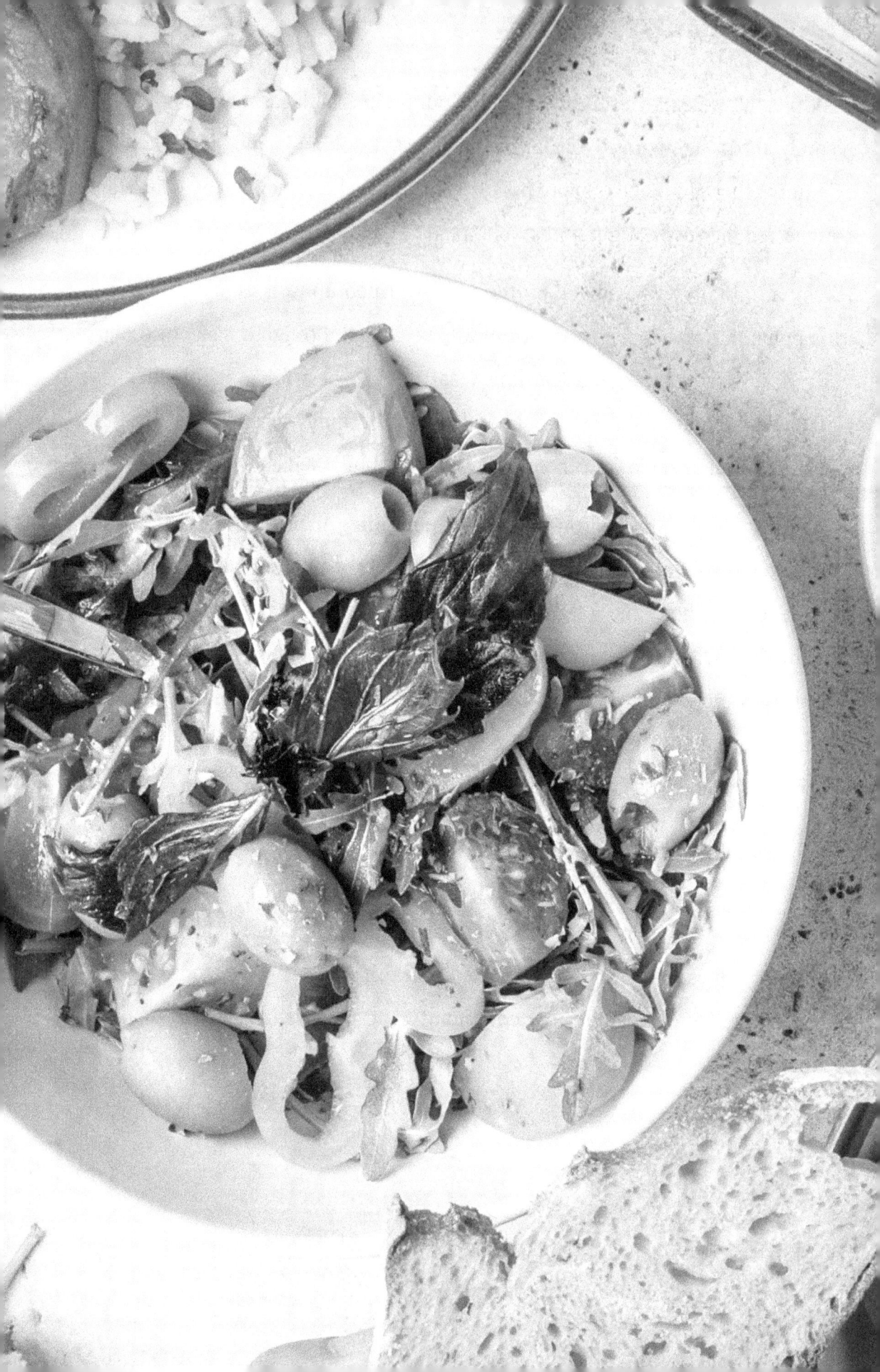

UNDERSTANDING YOUR GALLBLADDER

The Gallbladder's Role in Digestion

The human body is a marvel of biological engineering, and its digestive system is a testament to this complexity. This system is responsible for breaking down food into its most basic components, allowing our bodies to absorb nutrients, while discarding waste. Central to this process is a series of organs working in tandem, among which the gallbladder, although small, plays a pivotal role, especially in the digestion and absorption of fats. Nestled beneath the liver, the gallbladder acts as a storage unit for bile, a greenish-yellow fluid that the liver produces. The significance of the gallbladder may often be understated, but its role in our digestive health is undeniably important.

Situated on the inferior surface of the liver, the gallbladder is a small, pear-shaped organ that primarily functions as a bile reservoir. Bile is a critical digestive liquid produced by the liver, crucial for the digestion and absorption of fats. The gallbladder is connected to the liver and the small intestine via the biliary tract, comprising the cystic duct (connecting the gallbladder to the bile ducts) and the common bile duct (leading the bile into the small intestine). The gallbladder's ability to concentrate bile—by absorbing water and ions—makes the bile more effective in its digestive functions when released into the intestine.

The gallbladder's main function is to store and concentrate bile produced by the liver until it is needed for digesting fatty foods in the small intestine. When we consume fat-containing foods, the gallbladder contracts in response to signals from hormones such as cholecystokinin (CCK), releasing concentrated bile into the small intestine through the bile ducts. Bile salts emulsify fats in the digestive tract, breaking them down into smaller droplets. This action significantly increases the surface area of fats, making them more accessible to lipases, enzymes that further break down fats into fatty acids and glycerol. These products can then be absorbed by the intestinal lining into the bloodstream. Without the gallbladder's contribution, the digestion of fats would be less efficient, impacting nutrient absorption and overall health.

Despite its crucial role, the gallbladder is susceptible to several problems, primarily gallstones, which can obstruct the flow of bile, and cholecystitis, an inflammation of the gallbladder. Gallstones form when substances in bile, like cholesterol or bilirubin, harden. If they block the bile ducts, they can cause pain, nausea, and digestive issues, as the flow of bile into the intestine is impeded. Cholecystitis, often resulting from gallstones, leads to severe pain and, if left untreated, can affect the gallbladder's ability to function. In some cases, the removal of the gallbladder (cholecystectomy) is necessary. Although people can live without a gallbladder, this surgery can lead to changes in digestion, particularly in the process of digesting fats, requiring dietary adjustments.

Common Gallbladder Problems and Their Symptoms

The gallbladder, a small, pear-shaped organ located beneath the liver, plays a vital role in the digestive system. Its primary function is to store and concentrate bile, a fluid produced by the liver essential for the digestion and absorption of fats. Despite its importance, the gallbladder can be prone to various issues that significantly impact an individual's health and quality of life. Understanding common gallbladder problems, their symptoms, and potential complications is crucial for early detection and effective management.

Gallstones (Cholelithiasis)

Gallstones are the most common gallbladder issue, affecting millions worldwide. These are solid particles that form from bile cholesterol and bilirubin in the gallbladder. They range in size and can be as small as a grain of sand or as large as a golf ball. There are two types of gallstones: cholesterol stones, which are made mostly of hardened cholesterol and constitute about 80% of gallstones, and pigment stones, which are smaller and darker, made mostly from bilirubin.

Causes and Risk Factors: The exact causes of gallstones are not entirely understood, but several factors increase the risk, including gender (women are more prone), obesity, diet (high in fat and cholesterol, low in fiber), age (older individuals are at higher risk), and certain diseases and conditions that affect bile composition.

Symptoms and Complications: Many people with gallstones do not experience symptoms and may not require treatment. However, when symptoms occur, they can include sudden and intensifying pain in the upper right portion of the abdomen, back pain between the shoulder blades, and pain in the right shoulder. Nausea or vomiting may also accompany the pain. Complications can arise if gallstones block the flow of bile, leading to conditions such as cholecystitis (inflammation of the gallbladder), pancreatitis (inflammation of the pancreas), and jaundice.

Cholecystitis (Gallbladder Inflammation)

Cholecystitis is the inflammation of the gallbladder, often resulting from a gallstone blocking the cystic duct. It can be acute or chronic, with acute cholecystitis presenting a sudden onset of symptoms that can lead to severe complications if not treated.

Symptoms: Symptoms of acute cholecystitis include intense pain in the upper abdomen, fever, nausea, and vomiting. The pain may radiate to the back or right shoulder. Chronic cholecystitis may present with milder symptoms over a longer period, leading to a thickening of the gallbladder walls and a decrease in function.

Causes and Risk Factors: The primary cause of cholecystitis is the obstruction of the cystic duct by gallstones, leading to bile buildup and inflammation. Other risk factors mirror those of gallstones, including obesity, age, and diet.

Biliary Dyskinesia

Biliary dyskinesia is a condition characterized by abnormal muscle function of the gallbladder and bile ducts, leading to pain and digestive problems without the presence of gallstones. This condition is related to how the gallbladder empties bile.

Symptoms: The primary symptom is pain in the upper right abdomen, similar to gallstone pain, but without the presence of stones. Other symptoms include nausea, vomiting, and discomfort after eating, especially fatty meals.

Diagnosis and Treatment: Diagnosis involves tests to evaluate gallbladder function and ejection fraction. Treatment often includes dietary modifications to manage symptoms, and in some cases, surgical removal of the gallbladder may be recommended.

Gallbladder Cancer

Gallbladder cancer is a rare but serious condition. It is difficult to diagnose early because it often presents no specific symptoms until advanced stages.

Symptoms: When symptoms do appear, they may include abdominal pain, nausea, vomiting, bloating, and jaundice. These symptoms can easily be mistaken for those of less serious gallbladder issues, complicating early detection.

Risk Factors: Risk factors for gallbladder cancer include gallstones, chronic gallbladder inflammation, and certain genetic conditions. The presence of gallstones is a significant risk factor, although the majority of individuals with gallstones do not develop gallbladder cancer.

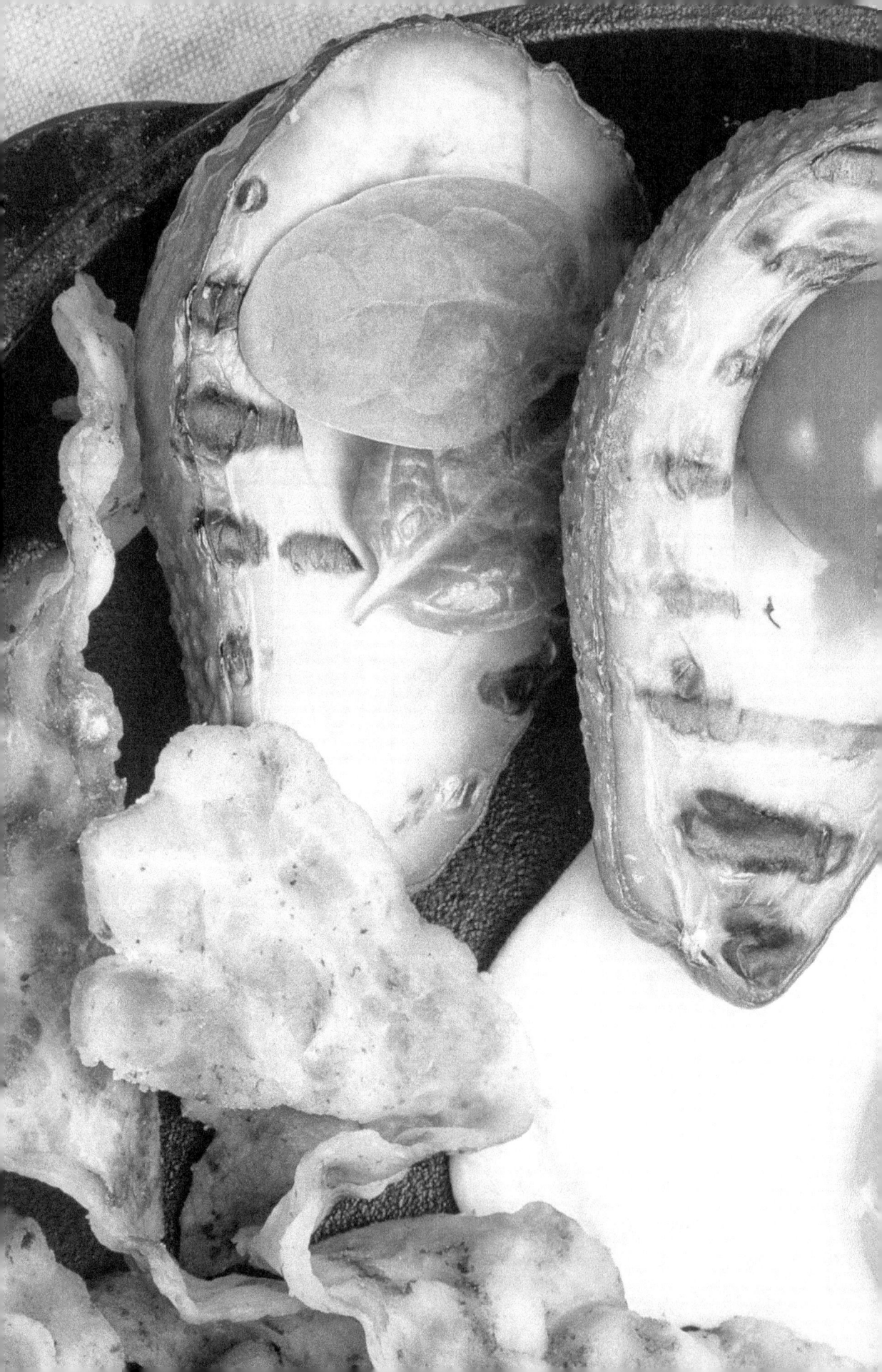

UNDERSTANDING THE GALLBLADDER DIET

Foods to Include for Gallbladder Health

In the realm of gallbladder health, the foods we choose to eat play a pivotal role. Incorporating high-fiber foods, healthy fats, and lean proteins into your diet can significantly improve gallbladder function and overall well-being.

Fiber is your digestive system's friend, especially when it comes to gallbladder health. Foods rich in fiber, such as fruits, vegetables, whole grains, and legumes, help regulate your digestive tract, ensuring everything moves smoothly. This smooth movement is crucial because it reduces the risk of gallstones, a common gallbladder issue. By incorporating a variety of fiber-rich foods into your diet, you're not only supporting your gallbladder but also enriching your body with essential nutrients that foster overall health.

Fiber Source	Portion Size	Calories (kcal)	Fiber (g)	Protein (g)	Fat (g)	Carbohydrates (g)
Oats	1/2 cup	150	4	5	2.5	27
Lentils	1/2 cup	115	7.8	9	0.4	20
Black Beans	1/2 cup	114	7.5	7.6	0.5	20.4
Chia Seeds	1 tbsp	58	5.5	3	3.7	5
Brussels Sprouts	1/2 cup	28	2	2	0.2	6
Avocado	1/4 medium	80	3.5	1	7	4

Pear (with skin)	1 medium	101	5.5	1	0.3	27
Apple (with skin)	1 medium	95	4	0.5	0.3	25
Raspberries	1/2 cup	32	4	0.7	0.4	7.3
Barley	1/2 cup	97	3	2	0.4	22
Quinoa	1/2 cup	111	2.6	4	1.8	19.7
Carrots	1/2 cup	25	1.7	0.6	0.1	5.8
Broccoli	1/2 cup	15	1.3	1.3	0.2	3
Sweet Potato	1/2 cup	90	3	2	0.2	21
Flaxseeds	1 tbsp	37	2.8	1.3	3	2
Almonds	1 oz	164	3.5	6	14.2	6.1
Peas	1/2 cup	62	4.4	4	0.2	11.1
Spinach	1/2 cup	3	0.7	0.4	0.1	0.6
Whole Wheat Bread	1 slice	69	1.9	3.6	1	11.6
Brown Rice	1/2 cup	108	1.8	2.5	0.9	22.4
Chickpeas	1/2 cup	134	6.2	7.3	2.1	22.5
Pears	1 medium	102	5.5	0.6	0.2	27.3

Apples	1 medium	95	4.4	0.5	0.3	25.1
Oranges	1 medium	62	3.1	1.2	0.2	15.4
Bananas	1 medium	105	3.1	1.3	0.4	27
Blueberries	1/2 cup	42	1.8	0.5	0.2	10.7
Strawberries	1/2 cup	24	1.5	0.5	0.2	5.8
Kale	1/2 cup	16	0.7	1.1	0.2	3.1
Beetroot	1/2 cup	37	1.7	1.4	0.1	8.5
Pumpkin Seeds	1 oz	158	1.7	8.5	13.9	1.8
Sunflower Seeds	1 oz	164	1.9	5.5	14	6.5
Walnuts	1 oz	185	1.9	4.3	18.5	3.9
Bok Choy	1/2 cup	10	0.7	1.1	0.1	1.5
Cabbage	1/2 cup	17	1.1	0.9	0.1	4
Cauliflower	1/2 cup	14	1.2	1.1	0.3	2.8
Mushrooms	1/2 cup	8	0.5	1.1	0.1	1.4
Zucchini	1/2 cup	9	0.6	0.6	0.1	1.9
Eggplant	1/2 cup	10	1.3	0.4	0.1	2.5

Tomatoes	1/2 cup	16	1.1	0.8	0.2	3.5
Cucumber	1/2 cup	8	0.3	0.3	0.1	1.9
Celery	1/2 cup	9	0.6	0.4	0.1	2
Asparagus	1/2 cup	13	1.5	1.5	0.1	2.5
Green Beans	1/2 cup	17	1.6	1	0.1	3.9
Artichokes	1/2 cup	45	4.5	2.2	0.1	10.5
Rye Bread	1 slice	83	2	2.5	1	15.5
Bulgur	1/2 cup	76	4.1	2.9	0.2	17
Farro	1/2 cup	100	3.5	3.5	0.5	26
Edamame	1/2 cup	95	4	8.5	4	7.5
Kiwi	1 medium	42	2.1	0.8	0.4	10.1

Healthy fats are another cornerstone of a gallbladder-friendly diet. Unlike their saturated counterparts, healthy fats — found in avocados, olive oil, nuts, and fatty fish like salmon and mackerel — support your heart and brain health without overburdening your gallbladder. Omega-3 fatty acids, in particular, are a type of healthy fat that can reduce inflammation and lower the risk of gallstones. Incorporating these fats into your meals can be as simple as dressing your salads with olive oil or snacking on a handful of walnuts.

Food Item	Portion Size	Fiber (g)	Total Fat (g)	Omega-3 (mg)	Calories
Avocado	1/2 medium	6.7	14.7	-	160
Chia Seeds	1 tbsp	4.1	4.4	2400	60
Flaxseeds	1 tbsp	2.8	4.3	1600	55
Walnuts	1 oz	1.9	18.5	2542	185
Almonds	1 oz	3.5	14.0	-	164
Olive Oil	1 tbsp	0	13.5	-	119
Ground Flaxseed Meal	1 tbsp	2.0	2.5	1200	37
Hemp Seeds	1 tbsp	0.9	4.7	1000	55
Pumpkin Seeds	1 oz	1.7	13.0	-	158
Sunflower Seeds	1 oz	1.5	14.0	-	164
Macadamia Nuts	1 oz	2.4	21.5	-	204
Pecans	1 oz	2.7	20.4	-	196
Brazil Nuts	1 oz	2.1	19.0	-	184
Sesame Seeds	1 tbsp	1.1	4.5	-	52
Coconut Oil	1 tbsp	0	13.5	-	117
Extra Virgin Olive Oil	1 tbsp	0	14.0	-	120
Canola Oil	1 tbsp	0	14.0	-	124
Soy Nuts	1 oz	3.0	6.0	-	130
Tofu (firm)	3.5 oz	2.3	8.7	-	124

Edamame	1/2 cup	4.0	8.0	-	120
Greek Yogurt (full-fat)	1 cup	0	9.0	-	190
Dark Chocolate (70-85% cacao)	1 oz	3.1	12.0	-	170
Salmon (wild-caught)	3 oz	0	10.5	2500	182
Trout (wild-caught)	3 oz	0	7.0	1000	128
Sardines (canned in water)	3.5 oz	0	10.5	1480	208
Chia Seed Oil	1 tbsp	0	14.0	7200	120
Flaxseed Oil	1 tbsp	0	14.0	7200	120
Walnut Oil	1 tbsp	0	14.0	1400	120
Avocado Oil	1 tbsp	0	14.0	-	124
Mackerel (wild-caught)	3 oz	0	17.0	4100	200
Herring (wild-caught)	3 oz	0	9.0	1700	134
Anchovies (canned in olive oil)	2 oz	0	10.0	1200	94
Cod Liver Oil	1 tsp	0	5.0	2700	45
Olive Tapenade	1 tbsp	0.5	7.0	-	80
Peanut Butter (natural)	2 tbsp	2.6	16.0	-	188
Cashew Butter	2 tbsp	0.9	14.0	-	165
Almond Butter	2 tbsp	3.3	18.0	-	202

Hazelnut Butter	2 tbsp	2.7	17.0	-	180		
Tahini (sesame seed paste)	1 tbsp	1.3	8.0	-	89		
Coconut Milk (light)	1/2 cup	0.5	5.0	-	50		
Spirulina	1 tbsp	1.0	1.0	-	20		
Seaweed	1 cup	0.3	0.5	-	9		

Lean proteins offer a gallbladder-safe alternative to fatty meats, which can exacerbate gallbladder issues. Lean meats like chicken, turkey, and fish, as well as plant-based proteins like lentils, beans, and tofu, provide the necessary building blocks for your body without the excess fat that can trigger gallbladder discomfort. By choosing lean proteins, you're ensuring that your body receives the protein it needs for repair and growth, all while maintaining gallbladder health.

Lean Protein Source	Fiber (g)	Portion Size	Calories	Protein (g)	Fat (g)	Sodium (mg)	Potassium (mg)
Chicken breast	0	3 oz	140	26	3	65	220
Turkey breast	0	3 oz	125	26	1	70	210
Egg whites	0	3 large	51	11	0	169	163

Cod	0	3 oz	70	15	0.5	60	439
Tofu (soft)	1	3 oz	70	8	4	10	150
Lentils	15.6	1 cup cooked	230	18	0.8	4	731
Chickpeas	12.5	1 cup cooked	269	14.5	4.2	11	477
Black beans	15	1 cup cooked	227	15	0.9	2	611
Greek yogurt (non-fat)	0	1 cup	100	17	0	61	240
Cottage cheese (low-fat)	0	1 cup	163	28	2.3	918	138
Quinoa	5.2	1 cup cooked	222	8	3.6	13	318
Edamame	8	1 cup	188	18	8	9	676
Salmon (wild)	0	3 oz	121	17	5.4	37	326
Tilapia	0	3 oz	110	22	2.5	85	302

Shrimp	0	3 oz	84	20	0.3	190	115
Peas	8.8	1 cup cooked	125	8	0.4	7	384
Almonds (skinless)	3.5	1 oz	163	6	14	0	200
Pumpkin seeds	1.7	1 oz	158	9	13	5	226
Flaxseeds	7.8	1 oz	150	5	12	8	230
Chia seeds	10.6	1 oz	138	4.7	8.7	5	115

Foods to Avoid

Navigating the dietary landscape for gallbladder health inevitably involves identifying and reducing the intake of high-fat and high-cholesterol foods. These types of foods can increase the risk of gallstone formation and lead to gallbladder attacks, marked by pain and discomfort.

High-fat foods, particularly those rich in saturated and trans fats, are found in many processed and fast foods, as well as in fatty cuts of meat and full-fat dairy products. These fats are not only harder for your gallbladder to process but also contribute to the buildup of cholesterol in your bile, increasing the likelihood of gallstones.

High-cholesterol foods can similarly impact your gallbladder health. While your body needs some cholesterol to function correctly, too much in your diet can lead to gallstones. Foods high in cholesterol include egg yolks, shellfish, and liver. Moderating your intake of these foods can help maintain a healthy gallbladder.

Reducing these types of foods in your diet doesn't mean sacrificing flavor or satisfaction. There are abundant healthy alternatives that can fill your plate. For instance, swapping out full-fat dairy for its low-fat or non-fat counterparts, choosing lean cuts of meat, and opting for cooking methods like baking, steaming, or grilling over frying can make a significant difference in your gallbladder health and overall dietary enjoyment.

Adapting Your Diet for Aging Digestive Systems

As we age, our digestive system undergoes changes that can affect how we process food. These changes make it essential to adapt our diet not only for gallbladder health but also to accommodate an aging digestive system. Modifying food textures and focusing on nutrient density can play a significant role in this adaptation.

Modifying textures of foods can aid in digestion and make eating a more pleasant experience. For those with chewing difficulties or reduced saliva production, softer foods like soups, stews, and smoothies can be both nutritious and easier to consume. Cooking methods that involve braising or stewing can transform tougher cuts of meat into tender, digestible meals, while blending fruits and vegetables into smoothies or soups can ensure you're still getting your daily dose of vitamins and minerals without the strain on your digestive system.

Focusing on nutrient density is crucial, especially for seniors who may eat less due to decreased appetite or other health issues. Nutrient-dense foods pack a high amount of vitamins, minerals, and other beneficial compounds into a small amount of food, ensuring that every bite counts. Incorporating foods like leafy green vegetables, berries, nuts, and seeds into your diet ensures you're getting a wide range of nutrients to support your body's needs without overloading your digestive system.

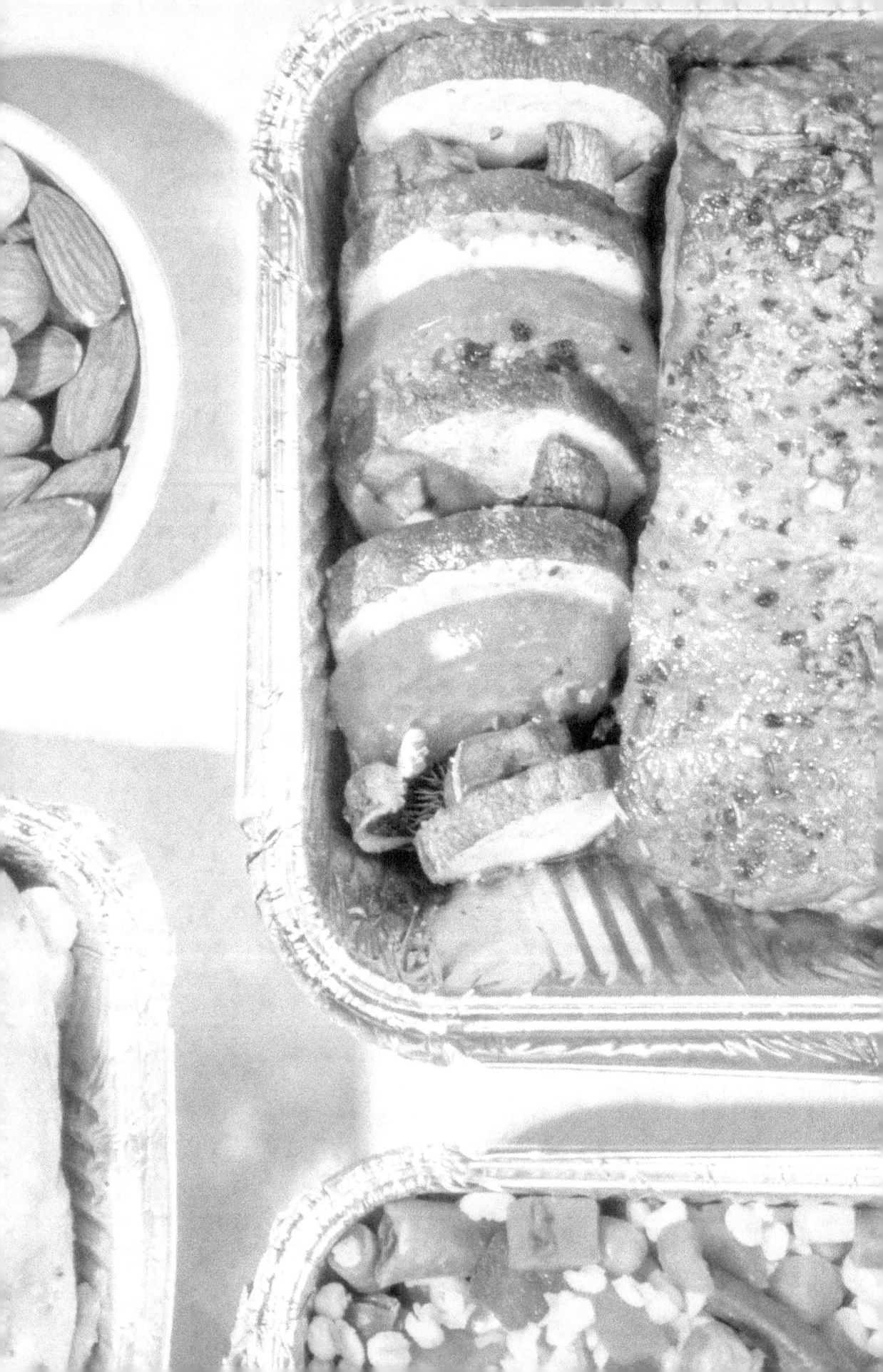

MEAL PLANNING AND PREPARATION

Shopping Lists and Meal Planning

A well-organized pantry and fridge are the cornerstones of a healthy diet, especially when managing gallbladder health. The process begins with purging items that are high in fats and low in nutritional value, replacing them with gallbladder-friendly alternatives like whole grains, lean proteins, and low-fat dairy products.

Creating a Master Shopping List: Start with a master list of ingredients that support gallbladder health, including fiber-rich fruits and vegetables, lean meats, and healthy fats from sources like fish and nuts. This list will serve as your guide, ensuring you always have the right ingredients on hand.

Meal Planning Strategies: Planning meals in advance can help you make healthier choices, reduce waste, and save money. Allocate some time each week to plan your meals, taking into account your nutritional needs and preferences. This can also be an excellent opportunity to explore new recipes that are both gallbladder-friendly and satisfying.

Organizing for Efficiency: Arrange your pantry and fridge in a way that makes healthy choices easy. Keep the most nutritious items at eye level, and organize your food by category, so you know exactly where everything is. This not only saves time but also makes it easier to stick to your gallbladder health goals.

Preparing Meals for One or Two

Cooking for one or two presents unique challenges, including the risk of food waste and the temptation to opt for less healthy convenience foods. However, with a few adjustments, you can enjoy homemade, nutritious meals that are just the right size.

Scaling Down Recipes: Learn to adjust recipes to suit your household size. This might mean halving or quartering ingredient amounts. There are many tools and apps available that can help you make these adjustments accurately, ensuring that your meals remain delicious and proportionate to your needs.

Smart Storage Solutions: Invest in quality storage containers that can keep leftovers fresh. Cooking a full recipe and then storing portions for later can save time and energy, providing you with ready-to-eat, healthy meals on demand.

Utilizing Ingredients Wisely: Plan meals that use overlapping ingredients to minimize waste. For example, if you buy a bag of spinach, you can use it in salads, omelets, and smoothies throughout the week. This approach ensures that you use what you buy, reducing waste and making meal prep more efficient.

Making Meal Prep Simple and Enjoyable

Meal prep doesn't have to be a chore. With the right strategies, you can make it a simple, enjoyable part of your routine that supports your gallbladder health and fits into your lifestyle.

Batch Cooking: One of the most efficient ways to prepare meals is to cook in batches. Set aside a few hours each week to prepare multiple meals that can be refrigerated or frozen. This not only saves time but also ensures that you have healthy options readily available.

Using the Right Tools: Equip your kitchen with tools that make meal prep easier. A good set of knives, a food processor, and slow cookers can significantly reduce prep time. These investments pay off in the long run by making cooking more enjoyable and less time-consuming.

Incorporating Fun into the Routine: Turn meal prep into a fun activity by involving family members or listening to your favorite music or podcasts while you cook. This can transform meal prep from a mundane task into a delightful part of your week.

Learning and Adapting: Be open to trying new recipes and techniques. The internet and cookbooks are full of ideas that can inspire your meal prep and introduce you to new, gallbladder-friendly foods and flavors. Embrace the learning process as part of the journey toward a healthier lifestyle.

By adopting these strategies under each subheading, you can enhance your approach to meal planning and preparation, making it a supportive pillar for gallbladder health and overall well-being.

LIFESTYLE CHANGES FOR GALLBLADDER HEALTH

Importance of Hydration

Hydration plays a critical role in maintaining gallbladder health. Adequate fluid intake helps to thin the bile, reducing the risk of gallstone formation. For seniors, staying well-hydrated is particularly important as the sensation of thirst may diminish with age, increasing the risk of dehydration.

How Much to Drink: The general recommendation is to drink at least eight 8-ounce glasses of water per day, but this can vary based on individual health, activity level, and climate. Including water-rich foods like fruits and vegetables in your diet can also contribute to your daily fluid intake.

Tips for Increasing Water Intake: Carry a reusable water bottle with you throughout the day to remind you to drink water regularly. Set reminders on your phone or watch as a prompt to take sips if you tend to forget to drink water. Herbal teas and infused water with slices of fruits or cucumbers can make hydrating more enjoyable without adding significant calories or sugar to your diet.

Monitoring Hydration Levels: Pay attention to the color of your urine as a quick hydration check. Light, straw-colored urine typically indicates good hydration, while dark yellow or amber-colored urine suggests you need to drink more water.

Exercise and Gallbladder Health

Regular physical activity is beneficial for overall health and can specifically aid in maintaining a healthy gallbladder by improving digestion and reducing the risk of gallstones. For seniors, finding safe and effective ways to stay active is key to reaping these benefits without risking injury.

Types of Recommended Activities: Low-impact exercises such as walking, swimming, cycling, and tai chi are excellent options for seniors. These activities can improve cardiovascular health, enhance flexibility, and strengthen muscles with a lower risk of stress on joints.

Creating a Balanced Routine: Aim for a mix of aerobic, strength, flexibility, and balance exercises to cover all aspects of physical fitness. Incorporating variety into your exercise routine can prevent boredom and promote a more comprehensive approach to health.

Consulting with Healthcare Providers: Before starting any new exercise program, it's important to consult with a healthcare provider, especially if you have existing health conditions. They can offer guidance on appropriate activities and intensity levels.

Stress Management and Sleep

Stress and poor sleep can adversely affect gallbladder health, contributing to issues like gallstone formation. Managing stress and prioritizing sleep are essential steps in creating a lifestyle that supports gallbladder health.

Techniques for Stress Reduction: Practices such as mindfulness meditation, deep-breathing exercises, and yoga can significantly reduce stress levels. Finding hobbies and activities that relax and engage you can also be a powerful antidote to stress.

Improving Sleep Hygiene: Establish a regular sleep schedule by going to bed and waking up at the same times every day, even on weekends. Create a relaxing bedtime routine to signal your body it's time to wind down. Keep your bedroom cool, dark, and quiet, and limit exposure to screens before bedtime to enhance sleep quality.

Seeking Professional Help: If stress or sleep issues persist despite your best efforts, consider seeking help from a mental health professional or sleep specialist. They can provide tailored strategies and support to address these challenges.

BREAKFAST RECIPE

Oatmeal with Almond and Pear

Prep Time: 5 minutes

Cooking Time: 10 minutes

Serving Size: 1 bowl

Ingredients:

- 1/2 cup rolled oats
- 1 cup almond milk
- 1 pear, diced
- 1 tablespoon almond slices
- 1 teaspoon honey
- 1/4 teaspoon cinnamon

Instructions:

1. Combine oats and almond milk in a small saucepan and bring to a boil. Reduce heat to low and simmer, stirring occasionally, until the oats are soft, about 5 minutes.
2. Stir in diced pear, almond slices, honey, and cinnamon. Cook for another 2-3 minutes, or until the pear is soft.
3. Serve warm.

Nutritional Information (per serving):

- Calories: 235.4
- Protein: 5.8g
- Sodium: 91mg
- Potassium: 258mg
- Total Fat: 4.8g
- Saturated Fat: 0.4g

- Cholesterol: 0mg
- Carbohydrates: 43.8g
- Fiber: 6.8g
- Sugars: 16.8g

Scrambled Tofu with Spinach and Tomatoes

Prep Time: 10 minutes

Cooking Time: 10 minutes

Serving Size: 1 serving

Ingredients:

- 1/2 block firm tofu, drained and crumbled
- 1 cup spinach, fresh
- 1/2 cup cherry tomatoes, halved
- 1 tablespoon olive oil
- Salt and pepper to taste
- 1/4 teaspoon turmeric for color

Instructions:

1. Heat olive oil in a skillet over medium heat. Add crumbled tofu and turmeric, sautéing for 5 minutes.
2. Add spinach and tomatoes, cooking until spinach is wilted and tomatoes are soft, about 5 minutes.
3. Season with salt and pepper. Serve hot.

Nutritional Information (per serving):

- Calories: 198.4
- Protein: 12.4g
- Sodium: 91.5mg
- Potassium: 259.4mg

- Total Fat: 14.4g
- Saturated Fat: 2.0g
- Cholesterol: 0mg
- Carbohydrates: 7.4g
- Fiber: 3.8g
- Sugars: 2.4g

Greek Yogurt with Honey and Mixed Berries

Prep Time: 5 minutes

Cooking Time: 0 minutes

Serving Size: 1 bowl

Ingredients:

- 1 cup low-fat Greek yogurt
- 1 tablespoon honey
- 1/2 cup mixed berries (strawberries, blueberries, raspberries)
- 1 tablespoon chopped walnuts

Instructions:

1. In a serving bowl, combine the Greek yogurt with honey.
2. Top with mixed berries and sprinkle with chopped walnuts.
3. Serve immediately for a refreshing and nutritious breakfast.

Nutritional Information (per serving):

- Calories: 245
- Protein: 20g
- Sodium: 55mg
- Potassium: 365mg
- Total Fat: 7g
- Saturated Fat: 1g

- Cholesterol: 10mg
- Carbohydrates: 28g
- Fiber: 3g
- Sugars: 24g

Avocado Toast with Poached Egg

Prep Time: 10 minutes

Cooking Time: 5 minutes

Serving Size: 1 serving

Ingredients:

- 1 slice whole-grain bread
- 1/2 ripe avocado
- 1 egg
- Salt and pepper to taste
- 1 teaspoon lemon juice
- Red pepper flakes (optional)

Instructions:

1. Poach the egg to your liking.
2. Mash the avocado with lemon juice, salt, and pepper.
3. Toast the whole-grain bread and spread the mashed avocado on top.
4. Place the poached egg over the avocado toast. Sprinkle with red pepper flakes if desired.
5. Serve immediately.

Nutritional Information (per serving):

- Calories: 310
- Protein: 13g
- Sodium: 210mg

- Potassium: 450mg
- Total Fat: 20g
- Saturated Fat: 4g
- Cholesterol: 185mg
- Carbohydrates: 22g
- Fiber: 7g
- Sugars: 3g

Smoothie Bowl with Spinach, Banana, and Flaxseed

Prep Time: 10 minutes

Cooking Time: 0 minutes

Serving Size: 1 bowl

Ingredients:

- 1 ripe banana
- 1 cup fresh spinach
- 1 tablespoon ground flaxseed
- 1/2 cup almond milk
- 1/2 cup mixed berries for topping
- 1 tablespoon unsweetened coconut flakes

Instructions:

1. Blend the banana, spinach, ground flaxseed, and almond milk until smooth.
2. Pour the mixture into a bowl.
3. Top with mixed berries and sprinkle with coconut flakes.
4. Serve immediately for a nutrient-packed breakfast.

Nutritional Information (per serving):

- Calories: 275

- Protein: 5g
- Sodium: 80mg
- Potassium: 600mg
- Total Fat: 7g
- Saturated Fat: 3g
- Cholesterol: 0mg
- Carbohydrates: 50g
- Fiber: 9g
- Sugars: 25g

Pear and Walnut Oatmeal

Prep Time: 5 minutes

Cooking Time: 15 minutes

Serving Size: 1 bowl

Ingredients:

- 1/2 cup rolled oats
- 1 cup water or almond milk
- 1 ripe pear, diced
- 1 tablespoon walnuts, chopped
- 1/4 teaspoon cinnamon
- 1 teaspoon honey or maple syrup (optional)

Instructions:

1. Cook the oats with water or almond milk according to package instructions.
2. Once the oatmeal is nearly done, stir in the diced pear and cinnamon. Cook for an additional 2 minutes.
3. Transfer to a bowl and top with chopped walnuts.

4. Drizzle with honey or maple syrup if desired.

5. Serve warm for a comforting breakfast.

Nutritional Information (per serving):

- Calories: 235
- Protein: 6g
- Sodium: 30mg
- Potassium: 200mg
- Total Fat: 5g
- Saturated Fat: 0.5g
- Cholesterol: 0mg
- Carbohydrates: 42g
- Fiber: 6g
- Sugars: 12g

Veggie and Herb Egg Muffins

Prep Time: 15 minutes

Cooking Time: 20 minutes

Serving Size: 1 muffin

Ingredients:

- 6 eggs
- 1/4 cup milk
- 1/2 cup spinach, chopped
- 1/4 cup bell peppers,
- diced
- 1/4 cup onions, diced
- 1 tablespoon fresh herbs (such as parsley or chives), chopped
- Salt and pepper to taste

- Non-stick cooking spray

Instructions:

1. Preheat the oven to 375°F and prepare a muffin tin with non-stick cooking spray.
2. In a large bowl, whisk together eggs, milk, salt, and pepper.
3. Stir in the spinach, bell peppers, onions, and fresh herbs.
4. Pour the egg mixture evenly into the muffin tin cups.
5. Bake for 20 minutes, or until the egg muffins are set and lightly golden on top.
6. Allow to cool slightly before serving.

Nutritional Information (per serving):

- Calories: 90
- Protein: 7g
- Sodium: 125mg
- Potassium: 125mg
- Total Fat: 6g
- Saturated Fat: 2g
- Cholesterol: 185mg
- Carbohydrates: 2g
- Fiber: 0.5g
- Sugars: 1g

Cinnamon Apple Quinoa Breakfast Bowl

Prep Time: 5 minutes

Cooking Time: 15 minutes

Serving Size: 1 bowl

Ingredients:

- 1/2 cup quinoa, rinsed
- 1 cup water
- 1 apple, diced
- 1/2 teaspoon cinnamon
- 1 tablespoon chopped almonds
- 1 teaspoon honey or maple syrup

Instructions:

1. In a small saucepan, combine quinoa and water. Bring to a boil, then reduce heat to low, cover, and simmer for about 15 minutes, or until quinoa is cooked and water is absorbed.
2. Stir in the diced apple and cinnamon during the last 5 minutes of cooking.
3. Transfer the cooked quinoa to a bowl. Top with chopped almonds and drizzle with honey or maple syrup.
4. Serve warm for a nutritious and comforting start to your day.

Nutritional Information (per serving):

- Calories: 290
- Protein: 8g
- Sodium: 10mg
- Potassium: 400mg
- Total Fat: 5g
- Saturated Fat: 0.5g

- Cholesterol: 0mg
- Carbohydrates: 55g
- Fiber: 6g
- Sugars: 15g

Spinach and Feta Breakfast Wrap

Prep Time: 10 minutes

Cooking Time: 5 minutes

Serving Size: 1 wrap

Ingredients:

- 1 whole grain tortilla
- 2 eggs, beaten
- 1/4 cup fresh spinach, chopped
- 2 tablespoons feta cheese, crumbled
- 1 tablespoon olive oil
- Salt and pepper to taste

Instructions:

1. Heat olive oil in a non-stick skillet over medium heat. Add beaten eggs and scramble until they are just set.
2. Stir in the chopped spinach and cook until wilted, about 1 minute. Season with salt and pepper.
3. Warm the whole grain tortilla in a separate pan or in the microwave for a few seconds.
4. Place the scrambled eggs and spinach mixture on the tortilla. Sprinkle with crumbled feta cheese.
5. Roll up the tortilla to enclose the filling. Serve immediately for a warm, savory breakfast wrap.

Nutritional Information (per serving):

- Calories: 320
- Protein: 18g
- Sodium: 420mg
- Potassium: 200mg
- Total Fat: 20g
- Saturated Fat: 6g
- Cholesterol: 370mg
- Carbohydrates: 20g
- Fiber: 3g
- Sugars: 2g

Berry Yogurt Smoothie

Prep Time: 5 minutes

Cooking Time: 0 minutes

Serving Size: 1 smoothie

Ingredients:

- 1/2 cup low-fat Greek yogurt
- 1/2 cup almond milk
- 1 cup mixed berries (strawberries, blueberries, raspberries)
- 1 banana
- 1 tablespoon chia seeds

Instructions:

1. In a blender, combine Greek yogurt, almond milk, mixed berries, banana, and chia seeds.
2. Blend on high speed until smooth and creamy.

3. Pour the smoothie into a glass and serve immediately for a refreshing and nutrient-packed breakfast.

Nutritional Information (per serving):

- Calories: 265
- Protein: 14g
- Sodium: 95mg
- Potassium: 550mg
- Total Fat: 4g
- Saturated Fat: 0.5g
- Cholesterol: 5mg
- Carbohydrates: 46g
- Fiber: 8g
- Sugars: 28g

SOUPS AND SALADS

Carrot Ginger Soup

Prep Time: 10 minutes

Cooking Time: 20 minutes

Serving Size: 1 cup

Ingredients:

- 1 tablespoon olive oil
- 1 onion, chopped
- 2 cloves garlic, minced
- 2 tablespoons fresh ginger, grated
- 1 pound carrots, peeled and diced
- 4 cups low-sodium vegetable broth
- Salt and pepper to taste
- Fresh parsley for garnish

Instructions:

1. Heat olive oil in a large pot over medium heat. Add onion and garlic, sautéing until softened, about 5 minutes.
2. Stir in the ginger and carrots, cooking for another 2 minutes.
3. Pour in the vegetable broth. Bring to a boil, then reduce heat and simmer until the carrots are tender, about 15 minutes.
4. Use an immersion blender to purée the soup until smooth. Season with salt and pepper.
5. Serve hot, garnished with fresh parsley.

Nutritional Information (per serving):

- Calories: 95
- Protein: 1.7g

- Sodium: 210mg
- Potassium: 360mg
- Total Fat: 3.5g
- Saturated Fat: 0.5g
- Cholesterol: 0mg
- Carbohydrates: 15g
- Fiber: 4g
- Sugars: 7g

Mixed Greens with Avocado and Citrus Dressing

Prep Time: 10 minutes

Cooking Time: 0 minutes

Serving Size: 1 salad

Ingredients:

- 2 cups mixed greens (spinach, arugula, and lettuce)
- 1/2 avocado, sliced
- 1/4 cup cherry tomatoes, halved
- 1/4 cucumber, sliced
- 2 tablespoons orange juice
- 1 tablespoon lemon juice
- 1 tablespoon olive oil
- Salt and pepper to taste
- 1 tablespoon slivered almonds

Instructions:

1. In a large bowl, combine the mixed greens, avocado slices, cherry tomatoes, and cucumber.

2. In a small bowl, whisk together orange juice, lemon juice, olive oil, salt, and pepper to create the dressing.

3. Drizzle the dressing over the salad and toss gently to coat.

4. Top the salad with slivered almonds.

5. Serve immediately for a fresh and nutritious meal.

Nutritional Information (per serving):

- Calories: 220
- Protein: 3g
- Sodium: 120mg
- Potassium: 720mg
- Total Fat: 19g
- Saturated Fat: 2.5g
- Cholesterol: 0mg
- Carbohydrates: 14g
- Fiber: 7g
- Sugars: 4g

Beetroot and Walnut Salad

Prep Time: 15 minutes

Cooking Time: 0 minutes

Serving Size: 1 salad

Ingredients:

- 2 medium beetroots, cooked and sliced
- 2 cups arugula
- 1/4 cup walnuts, chopped
- 2 tablespoons goat cheese, crumbled
- 2 tablespoons balsamic vinegar

- 1 tablespoon olive oil
- Salt and pepper to taste

Instructions:

1. Arrange the arugula on a serving plate. Top with sliced beetroots.
2. Sprinkle the chopped walnuts and crumbled goat cheese over the beets.
3. In a small bowl, whisk together balsamic vinegar, olive oil, salt, and pepper to create the dressing.
4. Drizzle the dressing over the salad just before serving.

Nutritional Information (per serving):

- Calories: 210
- Protein: 6g
- Sodium: 180mg
- Potassium: 400mg
- Total Fat: 16g
- Saturated Fat: 3g
- Cholesterol: 6mg
- Carbohydrates: 13g
- Fiber: 3g
- Sugars: 9g

Cucumber Tomato Feta Salad

Prep Time: 10 minutes

Cooking Time: 0 minutes

Serving Size: 1 salad

Ingredients:

- 1 large cucumber, diced
- 1 cup cherry tomatoes, halved

- 1/4 cup red onion, thinly sliced
- 1/4 cup feta cheese, crumbled
- 2 tablespoons olive oil
- 1 tablespoon lemon juice
- Salt and pepper to taste
- Fresh dill, chopped, for garnish

Instructions:

1. In a large bowl, combine cucumber, cherry tomatoes, and red onion.
2. Add crumbled feta cheese to the bowl.
3. In a small bowl, whisk together olive oil, lemon juice, salt, and pepper to make the dressing.
4. Pour the dressing over the salad and toss gently to combine.
5. Garnish with chopped fresh dill before serving.

Nutritional Information (per serving):

- Calories: 165
- Protein: 4g
- Sodium: 250mg
- Potassium: 350mg
- Total Fat: 14g
- Saturated Fat: 4g
- Cholesterol: 15mg
- Carbohydrates: 8g
- Fiber: 2g
- Sugars: 5g

Lemon Herb Chicken Soup

Prep Time: 10 minutes

Cooking Time: 30 minutes

Serving Size: 1 cup

Ingredients:

- 1 tablespoon olive oil
- 1 onion, chopped
- 2 carrots, peeled and diced
- 2 celery stalks, diced
- 2 cloves garlic, minced
- 4 cups low-sodium chicken broth
- 2 chicken breasts, cooked and shredded
- 1 lemon, zest and juice
- 1 teaspoon dried thyme
- Salt and pepper to taste
- Fresh parsley, chopped, for garnish

Instructions:

- Heat olive oil in a large pot over medium heat. Add onion, carrots, celery, and garlic. Sauté until vegetables are softened, about 5 minutes.
- Pour in chicken broth and bring to a boil. Reduce heat and simmer for 15 minutes.
- Add shredded chicken, lemon zest, lemon juice, and thyme to the pot. Season with salt and pepper.
- Cook for an additional 10 minutes, or until everything is heated through.
- Serve hot, garnished with fresh parsley.

Nutritional Information (per serving):

- Calories: 150
- Protein: 18g
- Sodium: 220mg
- Potassium: 360mg
- Total Fat: 4g
- Saturated Fat: 0.5g
- Cholesterol: 45mg
- Carbohydrates: 9g
- Fiber: 2g
- Sugars: 4g

Spinach Avocado Soup

Prep Time: 5 minutes

Cooking Time: 20 minutes

Serving Size: 1 cup

Ingredients:

- 1 tablespoon olive oil
- 1 onion, chopped
- 2 cloves garlic, minced
- 4 cups vegetable broth
- 4 cups spinach leaves
- 1 ripe avocado, peeled and pitted
- Salt and pepper to taste
- Lemon juice from 1 lemon

Instructions:

1. Heat olive oil in a large pot over medium heat. Add onion and garlic, sautéing until soft, about 5 minutes.

2. Add vegetable broth and bring to a boil. Reduce heat and simmer for 10 minutes.

3. Stir in spinach leaves, cooking until wilted, about 2 minutes.

4. Remove from heat and blend soup with an immersion blender until smooth.

5. Add avocado and lemon juice to the soup. Blend again until creamy.

6. Season with salt and pepper to taste. Serve warm.

Nutritional Information (per serving):

- Calories: 180
- Protein: 3g
- Sodium: 250mg
- Potassium: 550mg
- Total Fat: 15g
- Saturated Fat: 2g
- Cholesterol: 0mg
- Carbohydrates: 12g
- Fiber: 7g
- Sugars: 2g

Quinoa Vegetable Salad

Prep Time: 15 minutes

Cooking Time: 15 minutes

Serving Size: 1 salad

Ingredients:

- 1 cup quinoa, rinsed
- 2 cups water
- 1 cup cherry tomatoes, halved
- 1 cucumber, diced
- 1 bell pepper, diced
- 1/4 cup red onion, finely chopped
- 1/4 cup fresh parsley, chopped
- 3 tablespoons olive oil
- 2 tablespoons lemon juice
- Salt and pepper to taste

Instructions:

1. In a medium saucepan, combine quinoa and water. Bring to a boil, then cover, reduce heat to low, and simmer until quinoa is cooked and water is absorbed, about 15 minutes. Let cool.
2. In a large bowl, combine cooled quinoa, cherry tomatoes, cucumber, bell pepper, red onion, and parsley.
3. In a small bowl, whisk together olive oil, lemon juice, salt, and pepper to create the dressing.
4. Pour the dressing over the quinoa mixture and toss to combine.
5. Serve chilled or at room temperature.

Nutritional Information (per serving):

- Calories: 215

- Protein: 6g
- Sodium: 30mg
- Potassium: 320mg
- Total Fat: 10g
- Saturated Fat:
- Cholesterol: 0mg
- Carbohydrates: 28g
- Fiber: 4g
- Sugars: 3g

Broccoli Almond Soup

Prep Time: 10 minutes

Cooking Time: 20 minutes

Serving Size: 1 cup

Ingredients:

- 1 tablespoon olive oil
- 1 onion, chopped
- 2 cloves garlic, minced
- 4 cups vegetable broth
- 4 cups broccoli florets
- 1/4 cup almonds, toasted and chopped
- Salt and pepper to taste
- 1/4 cup low-fat milk or almond milk

Instructions:

1. Heat olive oil in a large pot over medium heat. Add onion and garlic, sautéing until translucent, about 5 minutes.

2. Add vegetable broth and broccoli florets. Bring to a boil, then reduce heat and simmer until broccoli is tender, about 15 minutes.

3. Use an immersion blender to purée the soup until smooth.

4. Stir in toasted almonds and milk. Season with salt and pepper to taste.

5. Heat through for an additional 2 minutes. Serve hot.

Nutritional Information (per serving):

- Calories: 140
- Protein: 5g
- Sodium: 260mg
- Potassium: 370mg
- Total Fat: 9g
- Saturated Fat: 1g
- Cholesterol: 0mg
- Carbohydrates: 12g
- Fiber: 4g
- Sugars: 3g

Tomato Basil Soup

Prep Time: 10 minutes

Cooking Time: 30 minutes

Serving Size: 1 cup

Ingredients:

- 1 tablespoon olive oil
- 1 onion, finely chopped
- 2 cloves garlic, minced
- 1 carrot, peeled and diced
- 4 cups low-sodium vegetable broth

- 2 cans (14.5 oz each) diced tomatoes, with juice
- 1/4 cup fresh basil, chopped
- Salt and pepper to taste
- 1/4 cup low-fat cream (optional for creaminess)

Instructions:

1. Heat olive oil in a large pot over medium heat. Add the onion, garlic, and carrot, sautéing until the vegetables are softened, about 5 minutes.
2. Add the vegetable broth and diced tomatoes with their juice. Bring to a boil, then reduce the heat and simmer for 20 minutes.
3. Stir in the chopped basil and continue to simmer for another 5 minutes.
4. Use an immersion blender to blend the soup until smooth. For a creamier texture, stir in low-fat cream at this point.
5. Season with salt and pepper to taste. Serve hot.

Nutritional Information (per serving):

- Calories: 90
- Protein: 2g
- Sodium: 290mg
- Potassium: 360mg
- Total Fat: 4g
- Saturated Fat: 1g (without cream)
- Cholesterol: 5mg (without cream)
- Carbohydrates: 12g
- Fiber: 3g
- Sugars: 6g

Arugula Pear Salad with Lemon Vinaigrette

Prep Time: 10 minutes

Cooking Time: 0 minutes

Serving Size: 1 salad

Ingredients:

- 2 cups arugula
- 1 pear, thinly sliced
- 1/4 cup walnuts, toasted and chopped
- 1/4 cup crumbled feta cheese
- 2 tablespoons olive oil
- 1 tablespoon lemon juice
- 1 teaspoon honey
- Salt and pepper to taste

Instructions:

1. In a large salad bowl, combine the arugula, sliced pear, toasted walnuts, and crumbled feta cheese.
2. In a small bowl, whisk together the olive oil, lemon juice, honey, salt, and pepper to create the lemon vinaigrette.
3. Drizzle the vinaigrette over the salad and toss gently to coat all the ingredients.
4. Serve immediately, offering a refreshing and nutritious salad with a delightful mix of flavors and textures.

Nutritional Information (per serving):

- Calories: 225
- Protein: 6g
- Sodium: 320mg
- Potassium: 250mg

- Total Fat: 18g
- Saturated Fat: 4g
- Cholesterol: 15mg
- Carbohydrates: 14g
- Fiber: 3g
- Sugars: 9g

MAIN DISHES

Baked Lemon Garlic Salmon

Prep Time: 10 minutes

Cooking Time: 20 minutes

Serving Size: 1 fillet

Ingredients:

- 4 salmon fillets (6 ounces each)
- 2 tablespoons olive oil
- 2 cloves garlic, minced
- 1 lemon, juice and zest
- 1 teaspoon dried dill
- Salt and pepper to taste
- Lemon slices for garnish

Instructions:

1. Preheat oven to 375°F. Line a baking sheet with parchment paper.
2. In a small bowl, mix together olive oil, garlic, lemon juice, lemon zest, dill, salt, and pepper.
3. Place salmon fillets on the prepared baking sheet. Brush each fillet with the lemon garlic mixture.
4. Bake for 20 minutes, or until salmon flakes easily with a fork.
5. Garnish with lemon slices before serving.

Nutritional Information (per serving):

- Calories: 280
- Protein: 23g
- Sodium: 75mg
- Potassium: 500mg

- Total Fat: 20g
- Saturated Fat: 3g
- Cholesterol: 60mg
- Carbohydrates: 2g
- Fiber: 0.5g
- Sugars: 0.5g

Quinoa Stuffed Bell Peppers

Prep Time: 15 minutes

Cooking Time: 30 minutes

Serving Size: 1 stuffed pepper

Ingredients:

- 4 large bell peppers, tops cut off and seeds removed
- 1 cup quinoa, cooked
- 1 tablespoon olive oil
- 1 onion, diced
- 2 cloves garlic, minced
- 1 zucchini, diced
- 1 cup spinach, chopped
- 1 tomato, diced
- 1/4 cup feta cheese, crumbled
- Salt and pepper to taste
- 1 teaspoon dried oregano

Instructions:

1. Preheat oven to 350°F. Place the bell peppers in a baking dish.
2. Heat olive oil in a skillet over medium heat. Add onion and garlic, cooking until soft.

3. Add zucchini and cook for another 5 minutes. Stir in spinach and tomato, cooking until the spinach is wilted.

4. Remove from heat and mix in the cooked quinoa, feta cheese, salt, pepper, and oregano.

5. Stuff each bell pepper with the quinoa mixture. Bake for 30 minutes.

6. Serve warm.

Nutritional Information (per serving):

- Calories: 220
- Protein: 8g
- Sodium: 180mg
- Potassium: 520mg
- Total Fat: 7g
- Saturated Fat: 2g
- Cholesterol: 8mg
- Carbohydrates: 34g
- Fiber: 6g
- Sugars: 8g

Grilled Chicken with Herbed Quinoa

Prep Time: 15 minutes (plus marination time)

Cooking Time: 20 minutes

Serving Size: 1 serving

Ingredients:

- 4 chicken breasts (6 ounces each)
- 2 tablespoons olive oil
- 1 lemon, juice and zest
- 2 cloves garlic, minced

- 1 teaspoon each of dried thyme, oregano, and rosemary
- Salt and pepper to taste
- 1 cup quinoa, cooked
- 1/4 cup fresh parsley, chopped

Instructions:

1. In a bowl, mix olive oil, lemon juice, lemon zest, garlic, thyme, oregano, rosemary, salt, and pepper. Marinate chicken breasts for at least 1 hour in the refrigerator.

2. Preheat grill to medium-high heat. Grill chicken for 10 minutes on each side or until fully cooked.

3. Toss cooked quinoa with chopped parsley. Season with salt and pepper.

4. Serve grilled chicken over herbed quinoa.

Nutritional Information (per serving):

- Calories: 360
- Protein: 35g
- Sodium: 85mg
- Potassium: 610mg
- Total Fat: 12g
- Saturated Fat: 2g
- Cholesterol: 90mg
- Carbohydrates: 28g
- Fiber: 4g
- Sugars: 1g

Turkey and Vegetable Skillet

Prep Time: 10 minutes

Cooking Time: 20 minutes

Serving Size: 1 serving

Ingredients:

- 1 tablespoon olive oil
- 1 pound ground turkey
- 1 onion, diced
- 2 cloves garlic, minced
- 1 zucchini, diced
- 1 bell pepper, diced
- 1 tomato, diced
- 1 teaspoon smoked paprika
- Salt and pepper to taste
- Fresh parsley, chopped, for garnish

Instructions:

1. Heat olive oil in a large skillet over medium heat. Add ground turkey, breaking it apart with a spatula. Cook until browned.
2. Add onion and garlic to the skillet. Cook until softened, about 5 minutes.
3. Stir in zucchini, bell pepper, and tomato. Season with smoked paprika, salt, and pepper. Cook until vegetables are tender, about 10 minutes.
4. Garnish with fresh parsley before serving.

Nutritional Information (per serving):

- Calories: 260
- Protein: 27g
- Sodium: 70mg

- Potassium: 650mg
- Total Fat: 14g
- Saturated Fat: 3g
- Cholesterol: 80mg
- Carbohydrates: 8g
- Fiber: 2g
- Sugars: 4g

Lemon Dill Baked Cod

Prep Time: 5 minutes

Cooking Time: 15 minutes

Serving Size: 1 fillet

Ingredients:

- 4 cod fillets (6 ounces each)
- 2 tablespoons olive oil
- 1 lemon, juice and zest
- 2 teaspoons fresh dill, chopped
- Salt and pepper to taste
- Lemon slices for garnish

Instructions:

1. Preheat oven to 400°F. Line a baking sheet with parchment paper.
2. Place cod fillets on the prepared baking sheet.
3. In a small bowl, mix together olive oil, lemon juice, lemon zest, dill, salt, and pepper.
4. Brush the mixture over the cod fillets.
5. Bake for 15 minutes, or until cod is flaky and cooked through.
6. Garnish with lemon slices and serve immediately.

Nutritional Information (per serving):

- Calories: 190
- Protein: 23g
- Sodium: 75mg
- Potassium: 460mg
- Total Fat: 10g
- Saturated Fat: 1.5g
- Cholesterol: 55mg
- Carbohydrates: 1g
- Fiber: 0g
- Sugars: 0g

Garlic Roasted Chicken and Vegetables

Prep Time: 15 minutes

Cooking Time: 35 minutes

Serving Size: 1 serving

Ingredients:

- 4 chicken thighs, skinless
- 1 tablespoon olive oil
- 4 cloves garlic, minced
- 1 teaspoon thyme, chopped
- 2 carrots, peeled and sliced
- 2 parsnips, peeled and sliced
- Salt and pepper to taste

Instructions:

1. Preheat oven to 425°F. In a large bowl, toss chicken thighs with olive oil, garlic, rosemary, thyme, salt, and pepper.

2. Arrange chicken, carrots, and parsnips on a baking sheet in a single layer.

3. Roast for 35 minutes, or until chicken is cooked through and vegetables are tender.

4. Serve hot, garnished with additional herbs if desired.

Nutritional Information (per serving):

- Calories: 310
- Protein: 24g
- Sodium: 85mg
- Potassium: 580mg
- Total Fat: 18g
- Saturated Fat: 4g
- Cholesterol: 110mg
- Carbohydrates: 12g
- Fiber: 3g
- Sugars: 5g

Spinach and Mushroom Quiche

Prep Time: 15 minutes

Cooking Time: 45 minutes

Serving Size: 1 slice

Ingredients:

- 1 pie crust (whole wheat for a healthier option)
- 1 tablespoon olive oil
- 1 onion, diced
- 2 cups mushrooms, sliced
- 2 cups spinach, chopped

- 4 eggs
- 1 cup low-fat milk
- 1/2 cup feta cheese, crumbled
- Salt and pepper to taste

Instructions:

1. Preheat oven to 375°F. Place pie crust in a pie dish.
2. Heat olive oil in a skillet over medium heat. Add onion and mushrooms, cooking until soft.
4. Add spinach and cook until wilted. Remove from heat and let cool.
5. In a bowl, whisk together eggs, milk, salt, and pepper.
6. Spread the vegetable mixture evenly over the pie crust. Sprinkle with feta cheese.
7. Pour the egg mixture over the vegetables and cheese.
8. Bake for 45 minutes, or until the quiche is set and the crust is golden.
9. Let cool for a few minutes before slicing and serving.

Nutritional Information (per serving):

- Calories: 220
- Protein: 10g
- Sodium: 320mg
- Potassium: 240mg
- Total Fat: 14g
- Saturated Fat: 5g
- Cholesterol: 110mg
- Carbohydrates: 15g
- Fiber: 2g
- Sugars: 3g

Ginger Soy Glazed Salmon

Prep Time: 10 minutes (plus marination time)

Cooking Time: 15 minutes

Serving Size: 1 fillet

Ingredients:

- 4 salmon fillets (6 ounces each)
- 1/4 cup low-sodium soy sauce
- 2 tablespoons honey
- 1 tablespoon fresh ginger, grated
- 2 cloves garlic, minced
- 1 tablespoon sesame oil
- 1 teaspoon rice vinegar
- Sesame seeds for garnish
- Green onions, sliced for garnish

Instructions:

1. In a small bowl, whisk together soy sauce, honey, ginger, garlic, sesame oil, and rice vinegar.
2. Place salmon fillets in a shallow dish and pour the marinade over them. Cover and refrigerate for at least 30 minutes.
3. Preheat oven to 400°F. Place salmon on a lined baking sheet and bake for 15 minutes, or until cooked through.
4. Garnish with sesame seeds and green onions before serving.

Nutritional Information (per serving):

- Calories: 295
- Protein: 23g
- Sodium: 320mg
- Potassium: 520mg

- Total Fat: 15g

- Saturated Fat: 2.5g

- Cholesterol: 60mg

- Carbohydrates: 12g

- Fiber: 0g

- Sugars: 10g

Mediterranean Vegetable Pasta

Prep Time: 15 minutes

Cooking Time: 20 minutes

Serving Size: 1 serving

Ingredients:

- 8 ounces whole wheat pasta

- 1 tablespoon olive oil

- 1 zucchini, sliced

- 1 bell pepper, diced

- 1/2 cup cherry tomatoes, halved

- 2 cloves garlic, minced

- 1/4 cup olives, sliced

- 1/4 cup low-sodium vegetable broth

- 1 teaspoon dried oregano

- Salt and pepper to taste

- 1/4 cup crumbled feta cheese

- Fresh basil for garnish

Instructions:

1. Cook pasta according to package instructions until al dente; drain and set aside.

2. In a large skillet, heat olive oil over medium heat. Add zucchini, bell pepper, cherry tomatoes, and garlic. Sauté until vegetables are tender, about 5-7 minutes.

3. Stir in olives, vegetable broth, oregano, salt, and pepper. Cook for an additional 3 minutes.

4. Toss the cooked pasta with the vegetable mixture. Heat through.

5. Serve topped with crumbled feta cheese and garnished with fresh basil.

Nutritional Information (per serving):

- Calories: 320
- Protein: 10g
- Sodium: 200mg
- Potassium: 370mg
- Total Fat: 9g
- Saturated Fat: 3g
- Cholesterol: 15mg
- Carbohydrates: 52g
- Fiber: 8g
- Sugars: 5g

Grilled Tilapia with Mango Salsa

Prep Time: 20 minutes

Cooking Time: 10 minutes

Serving Size: 1 fillet

Ingredients:

- 4 tilapia fillets (6 ounces each)
- 1 tablespoon olive oil
- Salt and pepper to taste

- 1 mango, diced
- 1/2 red bell pepper, diced
- 1/4 cup red onion, finely chopped
- 1 jalapeno, seeded and minced (optional)
- Juice of 1 lime
- 2 tablespoons cilantro, chopped
- Lime wedges for serving

Instructions:

1. Preheat grill to medium-high heat. Brush tilapia fillets with olive oil and season with salt and pepper.
2. Grill tilapia for about 4-5 minutes on each side, or until fish flakes easily with a fork.
3. In a bowl, combine mango, red bell pepper, red onion, jalapeno (if using), lime juice, and cilantro to make the salsa. Mix well.
4. Serve grilled tilapia topped with mango salsa. Accompany with lime wedges.

Nutritional Information (per serving):

- Calories: 250
- Protein: 23g
- Sodium: 85mg
- Potassium: 520mg
- Total Fat: 7g
- Saturated Fat: 1.5g
- Cholesterol: 55mg
- Carbohydrates: 18g
- Fiber: 2g
- Sugars: 12g

SNACKS AND LIGHT BITES

Avocado and Chickpea Salad Cups

Prep Time: 10 minutes

Cooking Time: 0 minutes

Serving Size: 1 cup

Ingredients:

- 1 ripe avocado, mashed
- 1/2 cup chickpeas, rinsed and drained
- 1 tablespoon lemon juice
- Salt and pepper to taste
- 1/4 teaspoon paprika
- 4 lettuce leaves (such as butter lettuce or romaine), to serve as cups
- 1 small tomato, diced
- 1 tablespoon chopped cilantro

Instructions:

1. In a bowl, mix together the mashed avocado, chickpeas, lemon juice, salt, pepper, and paprika until well combined.
2. Carefully spoon the avocado and chickpea mixture into the lettuce leaves, creating cups.
3. Top each cup with diced tomato and a sprinkle of chopped cilantro.
4. Serve immediately as a fresh and filling snack.

Nutritional Information (per serving):

- Calories: 150
- Protein: 4g
- Sodium: 15mg
- Potassium: 485mg

- Total Fat: 10g
- Saturated Fat: 1.5g
- Cholesterol: 0mg
- Carbohydrates: 12g
- Fiber: 7g
- Sugars: 2g

Cucumber Hummus Bites

Prep Time: 10 minutes

Cooking Time: 0 minutes

Serving Size: 1 bite

Ingredients:

- 1 large cucumber, sliced into rounds
- 1 cup hummus (preferably homemade or low-sodium)
- 1/4 cup red bell pepper, finely diced
- 1/4 cup carrot, finely diced
- 1 tablespoon sesame seeds
- Fresh parsley, for garnish

Instructions:

1. Lay the cucumber slices out on a serving platter.
2. Spoon a small amount of hummus onto each cucumber round.
3. Top each hummus-covered cucumber with a mixture of diced red bell pepper and carrot.
4. Sprinkle sesame seeds over the top for added texture and flavor.
5. Garnish with fresh parsley before serving as a crunchy and savory snack

Nutritional Information (per serving):

- Calories: 35
- Protein: 2g
- Sodium: 60mg
- Potassium: 115mg
- Total Fat: 2g
- Saturated Fat: 0.3g
- Cholesterol: 0mg
- Carbohydrates: 3g
- Fiber: 1g
- Sugars: 1g

Greek Yogurt and Berry Parfait

Prep Time: 5 minutes

Cooking Time: 0 minutes

Serving Size: 1 parfait

Ingredients:

- 1 cup low-fat Greek yogurt
- 1/2 cup mixed berries (strawberries, blueberries, raspberries)
- 2 tablespoons granola
- 1 teaspoon honey
- A sprinkle of cinnamon (optional)

Instructions:

1. In a serving glass or bowl, layer half of the Greek yogurt.
2. Add a layer of mixed berries on top of the yogurt.
3. Sprinkle 1 tablespoon of granola over the berries.
4. Repeat the layers with the remaining yogurt, berries, and granola.

5. Drizzle honey over the top and add a sprinkle of cinnamon if desired.

6. Serve immediately for a refreshing and nutritious snack.

Nutritional Information (per serving):

- Calories: 220
- Protein: 12g
- Sodium: 45mg
- Potassium: 240mg
- Total Fat: 3g
- Saturated Fat: 1g
- Cholesterol: 5mg
- Carbohydrates: 35g
- Fiber: 4g
- Sugars: 25g

Carrot and Hummus Roll-Ups

Prep Time: 10 minutes

Cooking Time: 0 minutes

Serving Size: 2 roll-ups

Ingredients:

- 2 large carrots, peeled
- 1/2 cup hummus
- 1/4 cup spinach leaves, finely chopped
- 1/4 cup red bell pepper, finely diced
- 1 tablespoon sesame seeds

Instructions:

1. Using a vegetable peeler, slice the carrots into long, thin strips.
2. Spread a thin layer of hummus over each carrot strip.

3. Sprinkle the chopped spinach and diced red bell pepper evenly over the hummus.

4. Carefully roll up the carrot strips.

5. Sprinkle sesame seeds over the roll-ups before serving.

Nutritional Information (per serving):

- Calories: 180
- Protein: 6g
- Sodium: 210mg
- Potassium: 320mg
- Total Fat: 8g
- Saturated Fat: 1g
- Cholesterol: 0mg
- Carbohydrates: 22g
- Fiber: 6g
- Sugars: 6g

Zucchini and Parmesan Crisps

Prep Time: 10 minutes

Cooking Time: 20 minutes

Serving Size: 1 serving (about 10 crisps)

Ingredients:

- 1 large zucchini, thinly sliced
- 1/4 cup grated Parmesan cheese
- 1 tablespoon olive oil
- Salt and pepper to taste

Instructions:

1. Preheat oven to 425°F. Line a baking sheet with parchment paper.

2. In a bowl, toss zucchini slices with olive oil, salt, and pepper.

3. Arrange zucchini slices in a single layer on the baking sheet.

4. Sprinkle grated Parmesan cheese over each slice.

5. Bake for 20 minutes, or until crispy and golden.

6. Serve immediately as a crunchy, savory snack.

Nutritional Information (per serving):

- Calories: 150
- Protein: 8g
- Sodium: 250mg
- Potassium: 450mg
- Total Fat: 10g
- Saturated Fat: 3g
- Cholesterol: 15mg
- Carbohydrates: 8g
- Fiber: 2g
- Sugars: 5g

Apple Peanut Butter Slices

Prep Time: 5 minutes

Cooking Time: 0 minutes

Serving Size: 1 serving (about 4 slices)

Ingredients:

- 1 apple, cored and sliced
- 2 tablespoons natural peanut butter
- 1 tablespoon chopped walnuts
- A sprinkle of cinnamon (optional)

Instructions:

1. Spread peanut butter evenly over the apple slices.

2. Sprinkle chopped walnuts over the peanut butter.

3. Add a sprinkle of cinnamon on top if desired.

4. Serve immediately for a sweet and crunchy snack.

Nutritional Information (per serving):

- Calories: 210

- Protein: 5g

- Sodium: 70mg

- Potassium: 250mg

- Total Fat: 12g

- Saturated Fat: 2g

- Cholesterol: 0mg

- Carbohydrates: 24g

- Fiber: 5g

- Sugars: 16g

Baked Sweet Potato Chips

Prep Time: 10 minutes

Cooking Time: 25 minutes

Serving Size: 1 serving (about 1 cup)

Ingredients:

- 1 large sweet potato, thinly sliced

- 1 tablespoon olive oil

- Salt and pepper to taste

- 1/2 teaspoon smoked paprika

Instructions:

1. Preheat oven to 400°F. Line a baking sheet with parchment paper.

2. Toss sweet potato slices with olive oil, salt, pepper, and smoked paprika until evenly coated.

3. Arrange slices in a single layer on the baking sheet.

4. Bake for 20-25 minutes, flipping halfway through, until crispy and edges are slightly browned.

5. Let cool before serving as a healthy, crunchy snack.

Nutritional Information (per serving):

- Calories: 140
- Protein: 2g
- Sodium: 120mg
- Potassium: 380mg
- Total Fat: 7g
- Saturated Fat: 1g
- Cholesterol: 0mg
- Carbohydrates: 18g
- Fiber: 3g
- Sugars: 5g

Pear and Ricotta Cheese Toast

Prep Time: 5 minutes

Cooking Time: 2 minutes

Serving Size: 1 toast

Ingredients:

- 1 slice whole-grain bread
- 2 tablespoons ricotta cheese
- 1/2 pear, thinly sliced
- 1 teaspoon honey
- A sprinkle of cinnamon (optional)

Instructions:

1. Toast the whole-grain bread to your liking.
2. Spread ricotta cheese evenly over the toasted bread.
3. Arrange thinly sliced pear on top of the ricotta.
4. Drizzle honey over the pear slices and add a sprinkle of cinnamon if desired.
5. Serve immediately for a sweet and satisfying snack.

Nutritional Information (per serving):

- Calories: 180
- Protein: 6g
- Sodium: 120mg
- Potassium: 150mg
- Total Fat: 4g
- Saturated Fat: 2g
- Cholesterol: 10mg
- Carbohydrates: 30g
- Fiber: 4g

- Sugars: 16g

Cucumber Avocado Rolls

Prep Time: 15 minutes

Cooking Time: 0 minutes

Serving Size: 1 roll

Ingredients:

- 1 large cucumber
- 1 avocado, mashed
- 1 tablespoon lime juice
- Salt and pepper to taste
- 1/4 cup carrot, julienned
- 1/4 cup red bell pepper, julienned
- Fresh cilantro for garnish

Instructions:

1. Using a vegetable peeler, slice the cucumber into long, thin strips.
2. In a small bowl, mix the mashed avocado with lime juice, salt, and pepper.
3. Lay out a cucumber strip and spread a thin layer of the avocado mixture near one end.
4. Place a few sticks of carrot and red bell pepper on top of the avocado.
5. Carefully roll the cucumber around the filling. Garnish with fresh cilantro.
6. Repeat with remaining cucumber strips and filling. Serve immediately as a fresh and crunchy snack.

Nutritional Information (per serving):

- Calories: 120

- Protein: 2g
- Sodium: 60mg
- Potassium: 360mg
- Total Fat: 9g
- Saturated Fat: 1.5g
- Cholesterol: 0mg
- Carbohydrates: 10g
- Fiber: 7g
- Sugars: 2g

Roasted Chickpeas with Herbs

Prep Time: 5 minutes

Cooking Time: 30 minutes

Serving Size: 1/4 cup

Ingredients:

- 1 can (15 oz) chickpeas, rinsed and drained
- 1 tablespoon olive oil
- 1/2 teaspoon garlic powder
- 1/2 teaspoon smoked paprika
- Salt and pepper to taste
- 1/4 teaspoon dried rosemary

Instructions:

1. Preheat oven to 400°F. Pat the chickpeas dry with paper towels.
2. In a bowl, toss chickpeas with olive oil, garlic powder, smoked paprika, salt, pepper, and dried rosemary until evenly coated.
3. Spread chickpeas in a single layer on a baking sheet.

4. Roast for 30 minutes, shaking the pan halfway through, until chickpeas are crispy and golden.

5. Let cool before serving as a crunchy, savory snack.

Nutritional Information (per serving):

- Calories: 150
- Protein: 5g
- Sodium: 200mg
- Potassium: 180mg
- Total Fat: 5g
- Saturated Fat: 0.7g
- Cholesterol: 0mg
- Carbohydrates: 20g
- Fiber: 6g
- Sugars: 3g

SMOOTHIES AND BEVERAGES

Anti-Inflammatory Turmeric Smoothie

Prep Time: 5 minutes

Cooking Time: 0 minutes

Serving Size: 1 smoothie

Ingredients:

- 1 banana, sliced and frozen
- 1/2 cup pineapple chunks
- 1 cup unsweetened almond milk
- 1/2 teaspoon turmeric powder
- 1/4 teaspoon ginger, grated
- A pinch of black pepper (to enhance turmeric absorption)
- 1 teaspoon honey (optional)

Instructions:

1. Place the banana, pineapple, almond milk, turmeric powder, ginger, and black pepper in a blender.
2. Blend on high until smooth and creamy. If the mixture is too thick, add a little more almond milk to reach your desired consistency.
3. Taste and add honey if a sweeter smoothie is preferred.
4. Serve immediately, enjoying the anti-inflammatory benefits of turmeric and ginger.

Nutritional Information (per serving):

- Calories: 185
- Protein: 2g
- Sodium: 90mg
- Potassium: 422mg

- Total Fat: 3g
- Saturated Fat: 0g
- Cholesterol: 0mg
- Carbohydrates: 40g
- Fiber: 5g
- Sugars: 25g

Green Detox Smoothie

Prep Time: 5 minutes

Cooking Time: 0 minutes

Serving Size: 1 smoothie

Ingredients:

- 1 cup fresh spinach
- 1/2 cucumber, sliced
- 1/2 apple, cored and sliced
- 1/2 cup frozen mango chunks
- 1 tablespoon chia seeds
- 1 cup coconut water
- Juice of 1/2 lemon

Instructions:

1. Combine spinach, cucumber, apple, mango, chia seeds, coconut water, and lemon juice in a blender.
2. Blend until smooth. If the smoothie is too thick, add more coconut water until you achieve the desired consistency.
3. Pour into a glass and serve immediately for a refreshing and detoxifying drink.

Nutritional Information (per serving):

- Calories: 160
- Protein: 3g
- Sodium: 25mg
- Potassium: 495mg
- Total Fat: 2.5g
- Saturated Fat: 0.5g
- Cholesterol: 0mg
- Carbohydrates: 34g
- Fiber: 6g
- Sugars: 25g

Berry Almond Milk Smoothie

Prep Time: 5 minutes

Cooking Time: 0 minutes

Serving Size: 1 smoothie

Ingredients:

- 1 cup mixed berries (strawberries, blueberries, raspberries), fresh or frozen
- 1 cup unsweetened almond milk
- 1 tablespoon almond butter
- 1 teaspoon flaxseed meal
- 1 teaspoon honey (optional)

Instructions:

1. Place the mixed berries, almond milk, almond butter, and flaxseed meal in a blender.
2. Blend on high until smooth. Add honey if a sweeter taste is desired.

3. Pour into a glass and serve immediately for a nutrient-packed, antioxidant-rich smoothie.

Nutritional Information (per serving):

- Calories: 200
- Protein: 4g
- Sodium: 180mg
- Potassium: 240mg
- Total Fat: 11g
- Saturated Fat: 1g
- Cholesterol: 0mg
- Carbohydrates: 24g
- Fiber: 6g
- Sugars: 15g

Cucumber Mint Water

Prep Time: 5 minutes

Cooking Time: 0 minutes

Serving Size: 1 glass

Ingredients:

- 1 cup cucumber, thinly sliced
- 2 tablespoons fresh mint leaves
- 1 liter of water

Instructions:

1. In a large pitcher, combine the cucumber slices, fresh mint leaves, and water.
2. Chill in the refrigerator for at least 1 hour to allow the flavors to infuse.

3. Serve cold, garnished with additional cucumber slices or mint leaves if desired.

Nutritional Information (per serving):

- Calories: 0
- Protein: 0g
- Sodium: 0mg
- Potassium: 76mg
- Total Fat: 0g
- Saturated Fat: 0g
- Cholesterol: 0mg
- Carbohydrates: 0g
- Fiber: 0g
- Sugars: 0g

Carrot Ginger Juice

Prep Time: 10 minutes

Cooking Time: 0 minutes

Serving Size: 1 glass

Ingredients:

- 4 large carrots, peeled
- 1 inch piece of ginger, peeled
- 1 apple, cored
- Juice of 1/2 lemon

Instructions:

1. Pass the carrots, ginger, and apple through a juicer.
2. Stir in the lemon juice to the extracted juice.

3. Serve immediately, or chill for an hour before serving for a refreshing, nutrient-dense juice.

Nutritional Information (per serving):

- Calories: 120
- Protein: 2g
- Sodium: 70mg
- Potassium: 410mg
- Total Fat: 0.5g
- Saturated Fat: 0g
- Cholesterol: 0mg
- Carbohydrates: 29g
- Fiber: 5g
- Sugars: 20g

Kiwi Spinach Smoothie

Prep Time: 5 minutes

Cooking Time: 0 minutes

Serving Size: 1 smoothie

Ingredients:

- 2 ripe kiwis, peeled and sliced
- 1 cup fresh spinach leaves
- 1 banana, sliced and frozen
- 1 cup unsweetened almond milk
- 1 tablespoon honey (optional)

Instructions:

1. Combine kiwis, spinach, banana, and almond milk in a blender.

2. Blend on high until smooth and creamy. Add honey for sweetness if desired.

3. Serve immediately for a vibrant, nutrient-rich smoothie.

Nutritional Information (per serving):

- Calories: 190
- Protein: 3g
- Sodium: 180mg
- Potassium: 650mg
- Total Fat: 3g
- Saturated Fat: 0g
- Cholesterol: 0mg
- Carbohydrates: 40g
- Fiber: 6g
- Sugars: 25g

Peach Basil Iced Tea

Prep Time: 5 minutes (plus chilling time)

Cooking Time: 10 minutes

Serving Size: 1 glass

Ingredients:

- 4 black tea bags
- 4 cups boiling water
- 2 peaches, sliced
- 1/4 cup fresh basil leaves
- Honey to taste (optional)

Instructions:

1. Steep the tea bags in boiling water for 5 minutes. Remove tea bags and let the tea cool to room temperature.

2. In a large pitcher, combine the brewed tea, peach slices and basil leaves.

3. Refrigerate until chilled, at least 1 hour.

4. Sweeten with honey if desired, stir well, and serve over ice.

Nutritional Information (per serving):

- Calories: 30
- Protein: 1g
- Sodium: 0mg
- Potassium: 150mg
- Total Fat: 0g
- Saturated Fat: 0g
- Cholesterol: 0mg
- Carbohydrates: 8g
- Fiber: 1g
- Sugars: 7g

Avocado Lime Smoothie

Prep Time: 5 minutes

Cooking Time: 0 minutes

Serving Size: 1 smoothie

Ingredients:

- 1 ripe avocado
- 1 cup spinach leaves
- Juice of 1 lime
- 1/2 cup coconut water

- 1/2 cup ice cubes
- 1 tablespoon honey (optional)

Instructions:

1. Scoop the avocado flesh into a blender and add the spinach leaves.
2. Pour in the lime juice and coconut water. Add the ice cubes.
3. Blend on high until smooth and creamy. Sweeten with honey if desired.
4. Serve immediately, enjoying the creamy texture and the refreshing taste of lime.

Nutritional Information (per serving):

- Calories: 230
- Protein: 3g
- Sodium: 30mg
- Potassium: 700mg
- Total Fat: 15g
- Saturated Fat: 2g
- Cholesterol: 0mg
- Carbohydrates: 26g
- Fiber: 10g
- Sugars: 12g

Watermelon Basil Hydrator

Prep Time: 5 minutes

Cooking Time: 0 minutes

Serving Size: 1 glass

Ingredients:

- 2 cups watermelon cubes
- 1/4 cup fresh basil leaves
- Juice of 1/2 lime
- 1/2 cup ice cubes
- Sparkling water (optional, for topping up)

Instructions:

1. Blend watermelon cubes, basil leaves, and lime juice together until smooth.
2. Add ice cubes and blend again briefly to chill the mixture.
3. Pour into a glass, optionally top up with sparkling water for a fizzy touch.
4. Serve immediately, garnished with a basil leaf or a slice of lime.

Nutritional Information (per serving):

- Calories: 60
- Protein: 1g
- Sodium: 0mg
- Potassium: 170mg
- Total Fat: 0g
- Saturated Fat: 0g
- Cholesterol: 0mg
- Carbohydrates: 15g
- Fiber: 1g

- Sugars: 12g

Ginger Pear Green Tea

Prep Time: 10 minutes (plus steeping time)

Cooking Time: 0 minutes

Serving Size: 1 glass

Ingredients:

- 1 green tea bag
- 1 cup hot water
- 1/2 pear, finely sliced
- 1 teaspoon grated ginger
- Honey to taste (optional)

Instructions:

1. Steep the green tea bag in hot water for 3-5 minutes, then remove the tea bag.
2. Add the sliced pear and grated ginger to the tea. Let it infuse for an additional 5 minutes.
3. Strain the mixture into a glass. Sweeten with honey if desired.
4. Serve warm, or chill in the refrigerator and serve over ice for a refreshing beverage.

Nutritional Information (per serving):

- Calories: 40
- Protein: 0g
- Sodium: 0mg
- Potassium: 95mg
- Total Fat: 0g
- Saturated Fat: 0g

- Cholesterol: 0mg
- Carbohydrates: 10g
- Fiber: 2g
- Sugars: 7g

Blueberry Almond Protein Shake

Prep Time: 5 minutes

Cooking Time: 0 minutes

Serving Size: 1 shake

Ingredients:

- 1 cup unsweetened almond milk
- 1/2 cup blueberries, fresh or frozen
- 1 scoop vanilla protein powder (ensure it's low in sugar and suitable for seniors)
- 1 tablespoon almond butter
- 1/2 banana, sliced
- 1/2 cup ice cubes

Instructions:

1. Place almond milk, blueberries, protein powder, almond butter, banana, and ice cubes in a blender.
2. Blend on high until smooth and creamy.
3. Pour into a glass and serve immediately for a nutritious, protein-rich snack.

Nutritional Information (per serving):

- Calories: 280
- Protein: 20g
- Sodium: 180mg

- Potassium: 400mg
- Total Fat: 10g
- Saturated Fat: 1g
- Cholesterol: 0mg
- Carbohydrates: 32g
- Fiber: 6g
- Sugars: 18g

DESSERTS

Baked Apple with Cinnamon and Walnuts

Prep Time: 10 minutes

Cooking Time: 30 minutes

Serving Size: 1 apple

Ingredients:

- 1 large apple, cored
- 2 tablespoons chopped walnuts
- 1/2 teaspoon ground cinnamon
- 1 teaspoon honey
- 1/4 cup water

Instructions:

1. Preheat your oven to 350°F (175°C).
2. Place the cored apple on a baking dish. Mix the chopped walnuts with cinnamon and stuff this mixture into the center of the apple.
3. Drizzle the honey over the stuffed apple.
4. Pour water into the bottom of the baking dish, around the apple, to help keep it moist while baking.
5. Bake in the preheated oven for about 30 minutes or until the apple is tender.
6. Serve warm, possibly with a dollop of low-fat yogurt if desired.

Nutritional Information (per serving):

- Calories: 180
- Protein: 2g
- Sodium: 0mg
- Potassium: 194mg

- Total Fat: 8g
- Saturated Fat: 1g
- Cholesterol: 0mg
- Carbohydrates: 27g
- Fiber: 5g
- Sugars: 20g

Mango Coconut Rice Pudding

Prep Time: 5 minutes

Cooking Time: 25 minutes

Serving Size: 1 cup

Ingredients:

- 1/2 cup Arborio rice or short-grain rice
- 1 can (14 oz) light coconut milk
- 1/4 cup water
- 2 tablespoons honey
- 1 ripe mango, diced
- 1/2 teaspoon vanilla extract

Instructions:

1. In a medium saucepan, combine the rice, light coconut milk, and water. Bring to a boil over medium heat.
2. Reduce the heat to low, cover, and simmer, stirring occasionally, until the rice is tender and the mixture is creamy, about 20 minutes.
3. Stir in the honey and vanilla extract, mixing well.
4. Remove from heat and let cool slightly. The pudding will thicken as it cools.
5. Just before serving, stir in the diced mango.

6. Serve warm or chilled, according to preference.

Nutritional Information (per serving):

- Calories: 220
- Protein: 3g
- Sodium: 30mg
- Potassium: 150mg
- Total Fat: 8g
- Saturated Fat: 7g
- Cholesterol: 0mg
- Carbohydrates: 36g
- **Fiber: 1g**
- **Sugars: 20g**

Raspberry Almond Chia Pudding

Prep Time: 10 minutes (plus chilling time)

Cooking Time: 0 minutes

Serving Size: 1 cup

Ingredients:

- 1/4 cup chia seeds
- 1 cup unsweetened almond milk
- 1 tablespoon honey or maple syrup
- 1/2 teaspoon vanilla extract
- 1/2 cup raspberries (fresh or frozen)
- 2 tablespoons slivered almonds

Instructions:

1. In a bowl, combine chia seeds, almond milk, honey (or maple syrup), and vanilla extract. Stir well.

2. Cover and refrigerate for at least 2 hours, or overnight, until it achieves a pudding-like consistency.

3. Before serving, top with raspberries and slivered almonds.

4. Enjoy as a refreshing and nutritious dessert or breakfast option.

Nutritional Information (per serving):

- Calories: 250
- Protein: 7g
- Sodium: 90mg
- Potassium: 200mg
- Total Fat: 14g
- Saturated Fat: 1g
- Cholesterol: 0mg
- Carbohydrates: 27g
- Fiber: 10g
- Sugars: 12g

Peach Yogurt Freeze

Prep Time: 5 minutes (plus freezing time)

Cooking Time: 0 minutes

Serving Size: 1 serving

Ingredients:

- 1 ripe peach, sliced
- 1 cup low-fat Greek yogurt
- 1 tablespoon honey
- A pinch of cinnamon

Instructions:

1. Blend the peach slices, Greek yogurt, honey, and cinnamon until smooth.

2. Pour the mixture into a shallow dish or ice cream molds.

3. Freeze for at least 4 hours or until firm.

4. Serve as a frozen treat, perfect for a hot day or as a healthy dessert option.

Nutritional Information (per serving):

- Calories: 180
- Protein
- Sodium: 55mg
- Potassium: 320mg
- Total Fat: 1g
- Saturated Fat: 0.5g
- Cholesterol: 8mg
- Carbohydrates: 27g
- Fiber: 2g
- Sugars: 25g

Dark Chocolate Avocado Mousse

Prep Time: 15 minutes

Cooking Time: 0 minutes

Serving Size: 1/2 cup

Ingredients:

- 1 ripe avocado
- 1/4 cup unsweetened cocoa powder
- 1/4 cup almond milk

- 2 tablespoons honey or maple syrup
- 1/2 teaspoon vanilla extract
- A pinch of salt

Instructions:

1. Blend the avocado, cocoa powder, almond milk, honey (or maple syrup), vanilla extract, and a pinch of salt in a food processor until smooth.
2. Refrigerate the mousse for at least 1 hour to thicken.
3. Serve chilled, garnished with a few berries or a sprinkle of cocoa powder if desired.

Nutritional Information (per serving):

- Calories: 200
- Protein: 3g
- Sodium: 75mg
- Potassium: 450mg
- Total Fat: 12g
- Saturated Fat: 2g
- Cholesterol: 0mg
- Carbohydrates: 25g
- Fiber: 7g
- Sugars: 15g

Baked Cinnamon Pears

Prep Time: 5 minutes

Cooking Time: 25 minutes

Serving Size: 1/2 pear

Ingredients:

- 2 ripe pears, halved and cored
- 2 teaspoons honey
- 1/2 teaspoon ground cinnamon
- 1/4 cup crushed walnuts

Instructions:

1. Preheat the oven to 350°F (175°C).
2. Place pear halves cut-side up on a baking sheet.
3. Drizzle each pear half with honey and sprinkle with cinnamon.
4. Top with crushed walnuts.
5. Bake for 25 minutes or until the pears are tender.
6. Serve warm, perhaps with a dollop of low-fat Greek yogurt.

Nutritional Information (per serving):

- Calories: 150
- Protein: 2g
- Sodium: 0mg
- Potassium: 175mg
- Total Fat: 7g
- Saturated Fat: 0.5g
- Cholesterol: 0mg
- Carbohydrates: 22g
- Fiber: 4g
- Sugars: 16g

Lemon Berry Sorbet

Prep Time: 10 minutes (plus freezing time)

Cooking Time: 0 minutes

Serving Size: 1/2 cup

Ingredients:

- 2 cups mixed berries (strawberries, blueberries, raspberries), fresh or frozen
- 1/4 cup fresh lemon juice
- 1/4 cup water
- 2 tablespoons honey or to taste

Instructions:

1. Blend the mixed berries, lemon juice, water, and honey in a blender until smooth.
2. Taste and adjust sweetness with more honey if needed.
3. Pour the mixture into a shallow dish and freeze until firm, about 4 hours.
4. Before serving, let the sorbet sit at room temperature for a few minutes to soften slightly.
5. Serve as a refreshing, light dessert.

Nutritional Information (per serving):

- Calories: 70
- Protein: 1g
- Sodium: 5mg
- Potassium: 85mg
- Total Fat: 0g

- Saturated Fat: 0g
- Cholesterol: 0mg
- Carbohydrates: 18g
- Fiber: 3g
- Sugars: 14g

Vanilla Almond Chia Seed Pudding

Prep Time: 10 minutes (plus chilling time)

Cooking Time: 0 minutes

Serving Size: 1 cup

Ingredients:

- 1/4 cup chia seeds
- 1 cup unsweetened almond milk
- 1 teaspoon vanilla extract
- 2 tablespoons maple syrup
- 2 tablespoons slivered almonds for topping

Instructions:

1. In a bowl, whisk together chia seeds, almond milk, vanilla extract, and maple syrup until well combined.
2. Cover the bowl with plastic wrap and refrigerate for at least 4 hours, or overnight, until it reaches a pudding-like consistency.
3. When ready to serve, give the pudding a good stir. If it's too thick, you can thin it with a little more almond milk.
4. Top with slivered almonds for added crunch and flavor.
5. Enjoy this simple yet delicious dessert that's perfect for a light snack or breakfast.

Nutritional Information (per serving):

- Calories: 240
- Protein: 6g
- Sodium: 95mg
- Potassium: 150mg
- Total Fat: 12g
- Saturated Fat: 1g
- Cholesterol: 0mg
- Carbohydrates: 29g
- Fiber: 10g
- Sugars: 14g

No-Bake Peanut Butter Oat Bars

Prep Time: 15 minutes (plus chilling time)

Cooking Time: 0 minutes

Serving Size: 1 bar

Ingredients:

- 1 cup rolled oats
- 1/2 cup natural peanut butter
- 1/4 cup honey
- 1/4 cup dark chocolate chips (optional)
- 1 teaspoon vanilla extract

Instructions:

1. In a large bowl, mix together the rolled oats, peanut butter, honey, and vanilla extract until well combined.
2. If using, fold in the dark chocolate chips.

3. Line a small baking dish with parchment paper and press the mixture firmly into the dish.

4. Refrigerate for at least 2 hours or until set.

5. Cut into bars and serve. These no-bake bars make a great dessert or snack that's easy to make and satisfying.

Nutritional Information (per serving):

- Calories: 180
- Protein: 5g
- Sodium: 75mg
- Potassium: 125mg
- Total Fat: 8g
- Saturated Fat: 2g
- Cholesterol: 0mg
- Carbohydrates: 24g
- Fiber: 3g
- Sugars: 12g

Grilled Pineapple with Honey Drizzle

Prep Time: 5 minutes

Cooking Time: 10 minutes

Serving Size: 1 slice

Ingredients:

- 4 pineapple slices, about 1/2-inch thick
- 2 tablespoons honey
- A pinch of ground cinnamon (optional)

Instructions:

1. Preheat the grill to medium-high heat.

2. Place pineapple slices on the grill and cook for about 5 minutes on each side, or until grill marks appear and the pineapple is heated through.

3. Drizzle honey over the grilled pineapple slices and sprinkle with a pinch of cinnamon if desired.

4. Serve warm as a delightful dessert that brings out the natural sweetness of pineapple.

Nutritional Information (per serving):

- Calories: 80
- Protein: 0g
- Sodium: 0mg
- Potassium: 120mg
- Total Fat: 0g
- Saturated Fat: 0g
- Cholesterol: 0mg
- Carbohydrates: 20g
- Fiber: 1g
- Sugars: 18g

FERMENTED FOODS FOR DIGESTIVE HEALTH

Homemade Sauerkraut

Prep Time: 20 minutes

Fermentation Time: 3 to 4 weeks

Serving Size: 1/4 cup

Ingredients:

- 1 medium head green cabbage (about 2 pounds)
- 1 tablespoon non-iodized sea salt

Instructions:

1. Remove the outer leaves of the cabbage and set aside. Slice the cabbage thinly.

2. In a large mixing bowl, combine the cabbage and sea salt. Massage the salt into the cabbage for about 5 to 10 minutes, until there is enough liquid to cover the cabbage.

3. Pack the cabbage tightly into a clean, sterilized jar, ensuring the liquid covers the cabbage completely to avoid exposure to air. Leave about an inch of space at the top.

4. Use one of the reserved outer leaves to cover the surface of the sauerkraut, tucking it down the sides of the jar to keep the shredded cabbage submerged.

5. Close the jar with a lid but not too tightly. If using a mason jar, consider a fermentation airlock lid to allow gases to escape.

6. Store the jar at room temperature, away from direct sunlight, for 3 to 4 weeks. Check periodically to ensure the cabbage remains submerged, pressing down if needed.

7. Taste the sauerkraut after 3 weeks. If it's to your liking, transfer the jar to the refrigerator to stop the fermentation process. It will keep for several months refrigerated.

Nutritional Information (per serving):

- Calories: 20
- Protein: 1g
- Sodium: 600mg
- Potassium: 70mg
- Total Fat: 0g
- Saturated Fat: 0g
- Cholesterol: 0mg
- Carbohydrates: 4g
- Fiber: 2g
- Sugars: 2g

Easy Kefir Yogurt

Prep Time: 10 minutes

Fermentation Time: 24 hours

Serving Size: 1 cup

Ingredients:

- 4 cups milk (preferably organic, whole or 2%)
- 1 packet kefir starter culture or 1 cup kefir from a previous batch

Instructions:

1. Gently warm the milk to room temperature or slightly above. Do not heat above 100°F to ensure the culture remains active.
2. If using a starter culture, follow the instructions on the packet to mix it with the milk. If using existing kefir, simply stir the kefir into the milk.

3. Transfer the mixture to a clean, sterilized jar. Cover loosely with a lid or a clean cloth secured with a rubber band.

4. Let the jar sit at room temperature, away from direct sunlight, for about 24 hours. The kefir will thicken and develop a tangy flavor as it ferments.

5. After 24 hours, taste the kefir. If it has reached your desired sourness, tighten the lid and refrigerate. If you prefer a stronger taste, let it ferment for a few more hours.

6. Stir the kefir well before serving. It can be enjoyed plain or with added fruits, honey, or nuts for flavor.

Nutritional Information (per serving):
- Calories: 150
- Protein: 8g
- Sodium: 100mg
- Potassium: 300mg
- Total Fat: 8g
- Saturated Fat: 5g
- Cholesterol: 20mg
- Carbohydrates: 12g
- Fiber: 0g
- Sugars: 12g

Ginger Beet Kvass

Prep Time: 15 minutes

Fermentation Time: 7 days

Serving Size: 1/2 cup

Ingredients:

- 3 medium beets, peeled and coarsely chopped
- 1 tablespoon grated ginger
- 1/4 cup whey (optional, for a quicker ferment)
- 1 tablespoon sea salt
- Filtered water, enough to fill a quart-sized jar

Instructions:

1. Place the chopped beets and grated ginger into a clean, quart-sized glass jar.
2. Add the whey (if using) and sea salt.
3. Fill the jar with filtered water, leaving about an inch of space from the top.
4. Stir to dissolve the salt and ensure the ingredients are well combined.
5. Cover the jar with a cloth and secure it with a rubber band or use an airlock lid.
6. Let the jar sit at room temperature, away from direct sunlight, for about 7 days.
7. Check the kvass daily, skimming off any foam or mold that may form on the surface.
8. After 7 days, taste the kvass. If it has a pleasing tart flavor, strain out the solids.
9. Transfer the kvass to the refrigerator in a clean bottle. Serve chilled.

Nutritional Information (per serving):

- Calories: 15
- Protein: 1g
- Sodium: 300mg
- Potassium: 87mg
- Total Fat: 0g
- Saturated Fat: 0g
- Cholesterol: 0mg
- Carbohydrates: 3g
- Fiber: 1g
- Sugars: 2g

Fermented Carrot Sticks

Prep Time: 15 minutes

Fermentation Time: 4-5 days

Serving Size: 2-3 sticks

Ingredients:

- 1 pound carrots, peeled and cut into sticks
- 2 cloves garlic, peeled
- 2 teaspoons sea salt
- 4 cups filtered water
- 2 dill sprigs (optional)

Instructions:

1. Dissolve the sea salt in the filtered water to make a brine solution.
2. Place the carrot sticks, garlic cloves, and dill sprigs into a clean, quart-sized glass jar.
3. Pour the brine over the carrots, ensuring they are completely submerged. Leave about an inch of space at the top of the jar.

106

4. If necessary, use a fermentation weight to keep the carrots submerged below the brine.

5. Cover the jar with a cloth and secure it with a rubber band, or use an airlock lid.

6. Let the jar sit at room temperature, away from direct sunlight, for 4-5 days.

7. Check daily, pressing down any carrots that rise above the brine.

8. Taste the carrots after 4 days. If they have a tangy flavor, transfer the jar to the refrigerator. Serve chilled.

Nutritional Information (per serving):

- Calories: 25
- Protein: 1g
- Sodium: 470mg
- Potassium: 200mg
- Total Fat: 0g
- Saturated Fat: 0g
- Cholesterol: 0mg
- Carbohydrates: 6g
- Fiber: 2g
- Sugars: 3g

Homemade Kimchi

Prep Time: 30 minutes

Fermentation Time: 1 week

Serving Size: 1/4 cup

Ingredients:

- 1 medium head Napa cabbage, chopped
- 1/4 cup sea salt
- Water, enough to cover cabbage
- 2 tablespoons grated ginger
- 4 cloves garlic, minced
- 2 teaspoons sugar
- 3 tablespoons fish sauce (optional)
- 1 tablespoon chili powder (adjust to taste)
- 1/2 cup julienned carrots
- 1/2 cup julienned daikon radish

Instructions:

1. Mix the chopped cabbage with sea salt and enough water to cover it in a large bowl. Let it sit for 2 hours, then rinse and drain.

2. Combine ginger, garlic, sugar, fish sauce (if using), and chili powder in a bowl to make the spice paste.

3. Add the drained cabbage to the spice paste along with julienned carrots and daikon. Mix thoroughly.

4. Pack the mixture into a clean, quart-sized jar, pressing down to eliminate air pockets and ensure the mix is submerged in its liquid.

5. Cover the jar with a cloth and secure with a rubber band or use an airlock lid.

6. Ferment at room temperature for 1 week, checking daily to ensure vegetables remain submerged.

7. Once fermented, store in the refrigerator. The kimchi will continue to ferment but at a slower pace.

Nutritional Information (per serving):

- Calories: 20
- Protein: 1g
- Sodium: 500mg
- Potassium: 60mg
- Total Fat: 0g
- Saturated Fat: 0g
- Cholesterol: 0mg
- Carbohydrates: 4g
- Fiber: 1g
- Sugars: 2g

Water Kefir

Prep Time: 10 minutes

Fermentation Time: 48 hours

Serving Size: 1 cup

Ingredients:

- 1/4 cup water kefir grains
- 1/4 cup sugar (cane sugar is preferred)
- 4 cups filtered water
- 1/2 lemon, sliced (optional)
- 2 dried figs (optional)

Instructions:

1. Dissolve the sugar in a small amount of hot water. Once dissolved, combine with the rest of the water in a quart-sized jar.

2. Add the water kefir grains to the jar along with lemon slices and dried figs if using.

3. Cover the jar with a cloth and secure it with a rubber band.

4. Let the mixture ferment at room temperature for 48 hours. The liquid should become slightly fizzy.

5. Strain out the kefir grains, lemon, and figs. The water kefir is now ready to drink. Store in the refrigerator.

6. The grains can be reused immediately for another batch or stored in the fridge in a small amount of sugar water.

Nutritional Information (per serving):

- Calories: 50
- Protein: 0g
- Sodium: 10mg
- Potassium: 20mg
- Total Fat: 0g
- Saturated Fat: 0g
- Cholesterol: 0mg
- Carbohydrates: 12g
- Fiber: 0g
- Sugars: 12g

Fermented Salsa

Prep Time: 20 minutes

Fermentation Time: 3-5 days

Serving Size: 1/4 cup

Ingredients:

- 4 medium tomatoes, diced
- 1 onion, finely chopped
- 2 jalapeños, minced (adjust to taste)
- 1/2 cup cilantro, chopped
- Juice of 1 lime
- 1 teaspoon sea salt
- 1/4 cup whey (optional, can help speed up fermentation)

Instructions:

1. Combine all ingredients in a bowl, mixing until well combined.
2. Pack the salsa mixture into a clean, quart-sized jar, leaving at least an inch of space at the top.
3. Press down firmly to ensure the salsa is submerged under its liquid.
4. Cover the jar with a cloth and secure with a rubber band or use an airlock lid.
5. Let the salsa ferment at room temperature for 3-5 days, checking daily to ensure it remains submerged.
6. Once fermented to your liking, place a tight lid on the jar and store in the refrigerator.

Nutritional Information (per serving):

- Calories: 15
- Protein: 1g
- Sodium: 200mg

- Potassium: 180mg
- Total Fat: 0g
- Saturated Fat: 0g
- Cholesterol: 0mg
- Carbohydrates: 3g
- Fiber: 1g
- Sugars: 2g

Fermented Garlic Honey

Prep Time: 10 minutes

Fermentation Time: 1 month

Serving Size: 1 teaspoon

Ingredients:

- 1 cup raw honey
- 1 head of garlic, cloves peeled

Instructions:

1. Place the peeled garlic cloves in a clean, pint-sized jar.
2. Pour the raw honey over the garlic cloves, ensuring they are completely covered. Leave some space at the top of the jar to allow for expansion.
3. Lightly cover the jar with a lid, allowing gases to escape, or use an airlock lid.
4. Store the jar at room temperature away from direct sunlight. Each day, open the jar to release any gases (this process is called "burping") and turn the jar upside down to ensure the garlic remains coated in honey.
5. After a month, the garlic will have fermented, infusing the honey with its flavor and beneficial properties. The garlic cloves can be eaten on

their own or used in cooking, and the honey can be used as a sweetener with added health benefits.

Nutritional Information (per serving):

- Calories: 60
- Protein: 0g
- Sodium: 0mg
- Potassium: 10mg
- Total Fat: 0g
- Saturated Fat: 0g
- Cholesterol: 0mg
- Carbohydrates: 17g
- Fiber: 0g
- Sugars: 16g

Cultured Cashew Cheese

Prep Time: 10 minutes (plus soaking time)

Fermentation Time: 24-48 hours

Serving Size: 2 tablespoons

Ingredients:

- 2 cups raw cashews, soaked in water for 4-6 hours then drained
- 1/4 cup rejuvelac or water kefir (for fermentation)
- 1/2 teaspoon sea salt
- 1 tablespoon nutritional yeast (optional, for a cheesy flavor)

Instructions:

1. After soaking, rinse the cashews and place them in a blender.
2. Add rejuvelac or water kefir, sea salt, and nutritional yeast if using. Blend until smooth and creamy.

3. Transfer the mixture to a clean, glass bowl. Cover with a cloth and secure with a rubber band.

4. Let the cashew mixture ferment at room temperature for 24-48 hours, depending on your taste preference and the room temperature.

5. Once fermented, stir the cheese, and it's ready to be enjoyed. Store in the refrigerator for up to a week.

Nutritional Information (per serving):

- Calories: 100
- Protein: 3g
- Sodium: 75mg
- Potassium: 125mg
- Total Fat: 7g
- Saturated Fat: 1.5g
- Cholesterol: 0mg
- Carbohydrates: 6g
- Fiber: 1g
- Sugars: 1g

Beet Kvass

Prep Time: 10 minutes

Fermentation Time: 7-14 days

Serving Size: 1/2 cup

Ingredients:

- 3 medium beets, peeled and coarsely chopped
- 1 tablespoon sea salt
- 4 cups filtered water

- 2 tablespoons whey or sauerkraut juice (optional, to kickstart fermentation)

Instructions:

1. Place the chopped beets in a clean, quart-sized glass jar.
2. Dissolve the sea salt in the filtered water and pour over the beets. Add whey or sauerkraut juice if using.
3. Ensure the beets are fully submerged by adding a fermentation weight or small glass jar.
4. Cover the jar with a cloth and secure with a rubber band or use an airlock lid.
5. Let the jar sit at room temperature, away from direct sunlight, for 7-14 days. Check periodically to ensure the beets remain submerged.
6. Taste the kvass after 7 days. If it has reached your desired level of tanginess, strain out the beets.
7. Store the beet kvass in the refrigerator. Serve chilled as a nutritious, probiotic-rich drink.

Nutritional Information (per serving):

- Calories: 20
- Protein: 1g
- Sodium: 350mg
- Potassium: 70mg
- Total Fat: 0g
- Saturated Fat: 0g
- Cholesterol: 0mg
- Carbohydrates: 4g
- Fiber: 1g
- Sugars: 3g

30-DAY MEAL PLAN

Day 1

- **Breakfast:** Oatmeal with Almond and Pear
- **Lunch:** Carrot Ginger Soup + Mixed Greens with Avocado and Citrus Dressing
- **Dinner:** Baked Lemon Garlic Salmon + Beetroot and Walnut Salad
- **Snacks:** Cucumber Hummus Bites
- **Beverage:** Anti-Inflammatory Turmeric Smoothie
- **Dessert:** Baked Apple with Cinnamon and Walnuts

Day 2

- **Breakfast:** Greek Yogurt with Honey and Mixed Berries
- **Lunch:** Lemon Herb Chicken Soup + Arugula Pear Salad with Lemon Vinaigrette
- **Dinner:** Quinoa Stuffed Bell Peppers
- **Snacks:** Avocado and Chickpea Salad Cups
- **Beverage:** Green Detox Smoothie
- **Dessert:** Mango Coconut Rice Pudding

Day 3

- **Breakfast:** Veggie and Herb Egg Muffins
- **Lunch:** Broccoli Almond Soup + Cucumber Tomato Feta Salad
- **Dinner:** Grilled Chicken with Herbed Quinoa
- **Snacks:** Greek Yogurt and Berry Parfait
- **Beverage:** Berry Almond Milk Smoothie
- **Dessert:** Raspberry Almond Chia Pudding

Day 4

- **Breakfast:** Avocado Toast with Poached Egg

- **Lunch:** Tomato Basil Soup + Beet Kvass
- **Dinner:** Turkey and Vegetable Skillet
- **Snacks:** Apple Peanut Butter Slices
- **Beverage:** Cucumber Mint Water
- **Dessert:** Peach Yogurt Freeze

Day 5

- **Breakfast:** Smoothie Bowl with Spinach, Banana, and Flaxseed
- **Lunch:** Spinach Avocado Soup + Beetroot and Walnut Salad
- **Dinner:** Lemon Dill Baked Cod
- **Snacks:** Baked Sweet Potato Chips
- **Beverage:** Carrot Ginger Juice
- **Dessert:** Dark Chocolate Avocado Mousse

Day 6

- **Breakfast:** Scrambled Tofu with Spinach and Tomatoes
- **Lunch:** Mixed Greens with Avocado and Citrus Dressing + Fermented Garlic Honey
- **Dinner:** Garlic Roasted Chicken and Vegetables
- **Snacks:** Pear and Ricotta Cheese Toast
- **Beverage:** Kiwi Spinach Smoothie
- **Dessert:** Baked Cinnamon Pears

Day 7

- **Breakfast:** Cinnamon Apple Quinoa Breakfast Bowl
- **Lunch:** Lemon Herb Chicken Soup + Arugula Pear Salad with Lemon Vinaigrette
- **Dinner:** Spinach and Mushroom Quiche
- **Snacks:** Cucumber Avocado Rolls
- **Beverage:** Peach Basil Iced Tea

- **Dessert:** Lemon Berry Sorbet

Day 8

- **Breakfast:** Pear and Walnut Oatmeal
- **Lunch:** Spinach Avocado Soup + Mixed Greens with Avocado and Citrus Dressing
- **Dinner:** Ginger Soy Glazed Salmon + Quinoa Stuffed Bell Peppers
- **Snacks:** Carrot and Hummus Roll-Ups
- **Beverage:** Avocado Lime Smoothie
- **Dessert:** Vanilla Almond Chia Seed Pudding

Day 9

- **Breakfast:** Spinach and Feta Breakfast Wrap
- **Lunch:** Broccoli Almond Soup + Cucumber Tomato Feta Salad
- **Dinner:** Mediterranean Vegetable Pasta
- **Snacks:** Greek Yogurt and Berry Parfait
- **Beverage:** Watermelon Basil Hydrator
- **Dessert:** No-Bake Peanut Butter Oat Bars

Day 10

- **Breakfast:** Berry Yogurt Smoothie
- **Lunch:** Tomato Basil Soup + Arugula Pear Salad with Lemon Vinaigrette
- **Dinner:** Grilled Tilapia with Mango Salsa
- **Snacks:** Avocado and Chickpea Salad Cups
- **Beverage:** Ginger Pear Green Tea
- **Dessert:** Grilled Pineapple with Honey Drizzle

Day 11

- **Breakfast:** Oatmeal with Almond and Pear
- **Lunch:** Carrot Ginger Soup + Beetroot and Walnut Salad

- **Dinner:** Baked Lemon Garlic Salmon + Greek Yogurt and Berry Parfait for a dessert-like snack
- **Snacks:** Baked Sweet Potato Chips
- **Beverage:** Kiwi Spinach Smoothie
- **Dessert:** Dark Chocolate Avocado Mousse

Day 12

- **Breakfast:** Scrambled Tofu with Spinach and Tomatoes
- **Lunch:** Lemon Herb Chicken Soup + Mixed Greens with Avocado and Citrus Dressing
- **Dinner:** Turkey and Vegetable Skillet
- **Snacks:** Cucumber Hummus Bites
- **Beverage:** Blueberry Almond Protein Shake
- **Dessert:** Baked Cinnamon Pears

Day 13

- **Breakfast:** Greek Yogurt with Honey and Mixed Berries
- **Lunch:** Spinach Avocado Soup + Cucumber Tomato Feta Salad
- **Dinner:** Garlic Roasted Chicken and Vegetables
- **Snacks:** Apple Peanut Butter Slices
- **Beverage:** Cucumber Mint Water
- **Dessert:** Raspberry Almond Chia Pudding

Day 14

- **Breakfast:** Veggie and Herb Egg Muffins
- **Lunch:** Broccoli Almond Soup + Beet Kvass
- **Dinner:** Spinach and Mushroom Quiche
- **Snacks:** Pear and Ricotta Cheese Toast
- **Beverage:** Peach Basil Iced Tea
- **Dessert:** Lemon Berry Sorbet

Day 15

- **Breakfast:** Cinnamon Apple Quinoa Breakfast Bowl
- **Lunch:** Tomato Basil Soup + Arugula Pear Salad with Lemon Vinaigrette
- **Dinner:** Quinoa Stuffed Bell Peppers
- **Snacks:** Cucumber Avocado Rolls
- **Beverage:** Green Detox Smoothie
- **Dessert:** No-Bake Peanut Butter Oat Bars

Day 16

- **Breakfast:** Berry Yogurt Smoothie
- **Lunch:** Lemon Herb Chicken Soup + Beetroot and Walnut Salad
- **Dinner:** Ginger Soy Glazed Salmon
- **Snacks:** Avocado and Chickpea Salad Cups
- **Beverage:** Peach Basil Iced Tea
- **Dessert:** Mango Coconut Rice Pudding

Day 17

- **Breakfast:** Scrambled Tofu with Spinach and Tomatoes
- **Lunch:** Broccoli Almond Soup + Mixed Greens with Avocado and Citrus Dressing
- **Dinner:** Garlic Roasted Chicken and Vegetables
- **Snacks:** Greek Yogurt and Berry Parfait
- **Beverage:** Berry Almond Milk Smoothie
- **Dessert:** Baked Apple with Cinnamon and Walnuts

Day 18

- **Breakfast:** Avocado Toast with Poached Egg
- **Lunch:** Spinach Avocado Soup + Cucumber Tomato Feta Salad
- **Dinner:** Mediterranean Vegetable Pasta

- **Snacks:** Carrot and Hummus Roll-Ups
- **Beverage:** Carrot Ginger Juice
- **Dessert:** Dark Chocolate Avocado Mousse

Day 19

- **Breakfast:** Smoothie Bowl with Spinach, Banana, and Flaxseed
- **Lunch:** Carrot Ginger Soup + Arugula Pear Salad with Lemon Vinaigrette
- **Dinner:** Grilled Tilapia with Mango Salsa
- **Snacks:** Baked Sweet Potato Chips
- **Beverage:** Kiwi Spinach Smoothie
- **Dessert:** Raspberry Almond Chia Pudding

Day 20

- **Breakfast:** Pear and Walnut Oatmeal
- **Lunch:** Tomato Basil Soup + Beet Kvass
- **Dinner:** Baked Lemon Garlic Salmon + Quinoa Stuffed Bell Peppers
- **Snacks:** Apple Peanut Butter Slices
- **Beverage:** Avocado Lime Smoothie
- **Dessert:** Peach Yogurt Freeze

Day 21

- **Breakfast:** Veggie and Herb Egg Muffins
- **Lunch:** Lemon Herb Chicken Soup + Mixed Greens with Avocado and Citrus Dressing
- **Dinner:** Turkey and Vegetable Skillet
- **Snacks:** Cucumber Hummus Bites
- **Beverage:** Watermelon Basil Hydrator
- **Dessert:** Lemon Berry Sorbet

Day 22

- **Breakfast:** Greek Yogurt with Honey and Mixed Berries
- **Lunch:** Spinach Avocado Soup + Arugula Pear Salad with Lemon Vinaigrette
- **Dinner:** Lemon Dill Baked Cod + Mixed Greens with Avocado and Citrus Dressing
- **Snacks:** Cucumber Avocado Rolls
- **Beverage:** Ginger Pear Green Tea
- **Dessert:** Vanilla Almond Chia Seed Pudding
- **Fermented Food:** Easy Kefir Yogurt (as part of breakfast or a snack)

Day 23

- **Breakfast:** Cinnamon Apple Quinoa Breakfast Bowl
- **Lunch:** Broccoli Almond Soup + Beetroot and Walnut Salad
- **Dinner:** Grilled Chicken with Herbed Quinoa
- **Snacks:** Carrot and Hummus Roll-Ups
- **Beverage:** Peach Basil Iced Tea
- **Dessert:** Grilled Pineapple with Honey Drizzle
- **Fermented Food:** Homemade Sauerkraut (added to the salad or as a side)

Day 24

- **Breakfast:** Berry Yogurt Smoothie
- **Lunch:** Lemon Herb Chicken Soup + Cucumber Tomato Feta Salad
- **Dinner:** Mediterranean Vegetable Pasta
- **Snacks:** Greek Yogurt and Berry Parfait
- **Beverage:** Kiwi Spinach Smoothie
- **Dessert:** No-Bake Peanut Butter Oat Bars

- **Fermented Food:** Cultured Cashew Cheese (as part of a snack or with dinner)

Day 25

- **Breakfast:** Pear and Walnut Oatmeal
- **Lunch:** Carrot Ginger Soup + Beet Kvass
- **Dinner:** Quinoa Stuffed Bell Peppers
- **Snacks:** Avocado and Chickpea Salad Cups
- **Beverage:** Cucumber Mint Water
- **Dessert:** Dark Chocolate Avocado Mousse
- **Fermented Food:** Ginger Beet Kvass (with lunch)

Day 26

- **Breakfast:** Smoothie Bowl with Spinach, Banana, and Flaxseed
- **Lunch:** Tomato Basil Soup + Mixed Greens with Avocado and Citrus Dressing
- **Dinner:** Turkey and Vegetable Skillet
- **Snacks:** Apple Peanut Butter Slices
- **Beverage:** Watermelon Basil Hydrator
- **Dessert:** Baked Cinnamon Pears
- **Fermented Food:** Water Kefir (as a beverage choice)

Day 27

- **Breakfast:** Veggie and Herb Egg Muffins
- **Lunch:** Spinach Avocado Soup + Arugula Pear Salad with Lemon Vinaigrette
- **Dinner:** Garlic Roasted Chicken and Vegetables
- **Snacks:** Baked Sweet Potato Chips
- **Beverage:** Avocado Lime Smoothie
- **Dessert:** Raspberry Almond Chia Pudding

- **Fermented Food:** Fermented Garlic Honey (on toast for a snack)

Day 28

- **Breakfast:** Oatmeal with Almond and Pear
- **Lunch:** Broccoli Almond Soup + Beetroot and Walnut Salad
- **Dinner:** Ginger Soy Glazed Salmon
- **Snacks:** Pear and Ricotta Cheese Toast
- **Beverage:** Anti-Inflammatory Turmeric Smoothie
- **Dessert:** Mango Coconut Rice Pudding
- **Fermented Food:** Homemade Sauerkraut (added to lunch)

Day 29

- **Breakfast:** Scrambled Tofu with Spinach and Tomatoes
- **Lunch:** Lemon Herb Chicken Soup + Cucumber Tomato Feta Salad
- **Dinner:** Baked Lemon Garlic Salmon + Quinoa Stuffed Bell Peppers
- **Snacks:** Cucumber Hummus Bites
- **Beverage:** Blueberry Almond Protein Shake
- **Dessert:** Peach Yogurt Freeze
- **Fermented Food:** Cultured Cashew Cheese (as part of a snack)

Day 30

- **Breakfast:** Avocado Toast with Poached Egg
- **Lunch:** Tomato Basil Soup + Mixed Greens with Avocado and Citrus Dressing
- **Dinner:** Mediterranean Vegetable Pasta
- **Snacks:** Greek Yogurt and Berry Parfait
- **Beverage:** Green Detox Smoothie
- **Dessert:** Lemon Berry Sorbet
- **Fermented Food:** Choose your favorite from the month (e.g., Easy Kefir Yogurt)

124

CONCLUSION

The "No Gallbladder Diet Cookbook and Food List for Seniors" represents a comprehensive guide designed to navigate the challenges of maintaining gallbladder health, particularly in the context of aging. This cookbook is not just a collection of recipes; it's a testament to adaptation, love, and the resilience of family bonds through culinary traditions. As we've explored the contents, the focus has been on understanding the gallbladder's crucial role in digestion, identifying foods that support its health while avoiding those that compromise it, and adapting diets to cater to the changing needs of an aging digestive system.

The meal planning and preparation section offered practical advice on organizing shopping lists, meal planning strategies, and tips for cooking for one or two, highlighting the importance of making meal prep simple and enjoyable. Lifestyle changes for gallbladder health emphasized hydration, exercise, stress management, and sleep, underlining the holistic approach needed to maintain overall well-being.

The recipes section provided a diverse range of gallbladder-friendly meals, from nutrient-packed breakfast options like Oatmeal with Almond and Pear, to hearty main dishes such as Baked Lemon Garlic Salmon, and even included snacks, smoothies, and desserts that cater to a healthy gallbladder diet. Each recipe was crafted with an eye towards balancing nutrition, ease of preparation, and flavor, ensuring that meals remain both satisfying and supportive of gallbladder and overall health.

Fermented foods were highlighted for their digestive health benefits, with simple recipes for Homemade Sauerkraut, Easy Kefir Yogurt, and Ginger Beet

Kvass, among others. These additions aim to introduce beneficial bacteria into the diet, supporting the digestive system and enhancing nutrient absorption.

The 30-day meal plan serves as a roadmap, offering a structured approach to integrating the principles and recipes from the cookbook into daily life. This plan emphasizes variety, nutritional balance, and the inclusion of fermented foods, ensuring a comprehensive approach to gallbladder health.

In conclusion, this cookbook goes beyond mere recipes; it serves as an educational resource, a practical guide, and a source of inspiration for seniors navigating the challenges of gallbladder health. It celebrates the power of food as a means of connection, healing, and joy. Through its pages, readers are encouraged to embrace change with creativity and courage, proving that a gallbladder-friendly diet can be both delicious and fulfilling, preserving the joy of eating without compromising on health.